Cultural Studies and Transdisciplinarity in Education

Series Editors
Aaron Koh
National Institute of Education, Nanyang Technological University, Singapore, Singapore

Victoria Carrington
School of Education & Lifelong Learning University of East Anglia, Norwich, United Kingdom

We live in a time where the complex nature and implications of social, political and cultural issues for individuals and groups is increasingly clear. While this may lead some to focus on smaller and smaller units of analysis in the hope that by understanding the parts we may begin to understand the whole, this book series is premised on the strongly held view that researchers, practitioners and policy makers interested in education will increasingly need to integrate knowledge gained from a range of disciplinary and theoretical sources in order to frame and address these complex issues. A transdisciplinary approach takes account the uncertainty of knowledge and the complexity of social and cultural issues relevant to education. It acknowledges that there will be unresolved tensions and that these should be seen as productive. With this in mind, the reflexive and critical nature of cultural studies and its focus on the processes and currents that construct our daily lives has made it a central point of reference for many working in the contemporary social sciences and education.

This book series seeks to foreground transdisciplinary and cultural studies influenced scholarship with a view to building conversations, ideas and sustainable networks of knowledge that may prove crucial to the ongoing development and relevance of the field of educational studies. The series will place a premium on manuscripts that critically engage with key educational issues from a position that draws from cultural studies or demonstrates a transdisciplinary approach. This can take the form of reports of new empirical research, critical discussions and/or theoretical pieces. In addition, the series editors are particularly keen to accept work that takes as its focus issues that draw from the wider Asia Pacific region but that may have relevance more globally, however all proposals that reflect the diversity of contemporary educational research will be considered.

Book proposals for this series may be submitted to the Publishing Editor: **Lawrence Liu**
E-mail: Lawrence.Liu@springer.com

More information about this series at http://www.springer.com/series/11200

Johannah Fahey • Howard Prosser • Matthew Shaw
Editors

In the Realm of the Senses

Social Aesthetics and the Sensory Dynamics of Privilege

Springer

Editors
Johannah Fahey
Faculty of Education
Monash University
Melbourne
Victoria
Australia

Matthew Shaw
Faculty of Education
Monash University
Melbourne
Victoria
Australia

Howard Prosser
Faculty of Education
Monash University
Melbourne
Victoria
Australia

ISSN 2345-7708 ISSN 2345-7716 (electronic)
Cultural Studies and Transdisciplinarity in Education
ISBN 978-981-287-349-1 ISBN 978-981-287-350-7 (eBook)
DOI 10.1007/978-981-287-350-7

Library of Congress Control Number: 2015933508

Springer Singapore Heidelberg New York Dordrecht London

Printed on acid-free paper

Springer is a brand of Springer Singapore
Springer is part of Springer Science+Business Media (www.springer.com)

Acknowledgements

We would like to express our gratitude to the Australian Research Council, which funded the 5 year Discovery-Project *Elite independent schools in globalising circumstances: a multi-sited global ethnography* (2010–2014). This book stems from that project. We would also like to thank the Faculty of Education, Monash University for providing the institutional base within which to write. Thanks to our contributing authors who worked tirelessly to produce chapters aimed at interrogating and developing our understandings of social aesthetics, and who all contributed immensely to the final product through their feedback, support and encouragement. We would also like to thank our publishing editor Lawrence Lui and our series editors Aaron Koh and Victoria Carrington, who facilitated the rigorous peer review process that greatly improved the overall quality of this book. We are also grateful to all the people who participated in our interviews and posed for our photos. We thank Hugh McLean for introducing us to David MacDougall's films, and David MacDougall for his generous involvement during our writing process. Tina 'swami' Inserra provided her valuable Photoshop skills and we express our sincere appreciation to her. The photograph of the Khayelitsha township in South Africa is courtesy of Chell Hill and we thank him for allowing us to use his image. Last, but not least, we offer enormous gratitude to our families for providing us with love and support during the process of assembling this book.

Contents

Contributors

Ergin Bulut University of Illinois at Urbana Champaign, Champaign, USA

Michelle Castro University of Illinois at Urbana Champaign, Champaign, USA

Johannah Fahey Monash University, Melbourne, Australia

Koeli Goel University of Illinois at Urbana Champaign, Champaign, USA

Heather Greenhalgh-Spencer Texas Tech University, Lubbock, TX, USA

Jane Kenway Monash University, Melbourne, Australia

Aaron Koh Nanyang Technological University, Singapore, Singapore

Chunfeng Lin University of Illinois at Urbana Champaign, Champaign, USA

David MacDougall Australian National University, Canberra, Australia

Cameron McCarthy University of Illinois at Urbana Champaign, Champaign, USA

Howard Prosser Monash University, Melbourne, Australia

Fazal Rizvi The University of Melbourne, Melbourne, Australia

Brenda Sanya University of Illinois at Urbana Champaign, Champaign, USA

Matthew Shaw Monash University, Melbourne, Australia

Introduction: Local Classes, Global Influences—Considerations on the Social Aesthetics of Elite Schools

Johannah Fahey, Howard Prosser and Matthew Shaw

Introduction (Fig. 1)

Imagine the sound of girls' whispered conversations, their countless footfalls echoing on wooden stairs that lead to a checkerboard marbled floor beneath a low-beamed wooden ceiling in a corridor of Highbury Hall. This institution is one of England's most privileged girls boarding schools, its first principal a suffragette dedicated to the cause of women's education.[1] Picture in your mind's eye boys (in trousers and long-sleeved shirts) and girls (in salwar kameez) formally attired and congregating for the twilight walk to the dining room of Ripon College, a school established during India's colonial British Raj to educate the rulers of India's princely states. The dusty paths are laden with the blush of heavy Bougainvillea, the air filled with the mournful cry of peacocks and punctuated by unceasing car-horns emanating from the pollution-riddled streets beyond. Visualize students hurrying through the grand and guarded entrance of the Straits School, a school originally conceived

[1] When we speak of 'privilege' it refers to the special entitlements that are granted to a restricted group, in this case those largely social, economic and political advantages that accrue for the students who attend these elite schools. We talk about the 'dynamics of privilege' to acknowledge that privilege is not necessarily a static or constant entity. Rather, there is a constant process of reinvention, adaptation and negotiation in relation to the entitlements granted to these elite schools and their students. One example of 'entitlement', which was witnessed across all the schools, is the belief (on behalf of the school administration, the student's parents and the students themselves) that no matter what these students do they will succeed. Of course, the counterpoint to such a belief is an apparent inability to deal with failure.

J. Fahey (✉) · H. Prosser · M. Shaw
Monash University, Melbourne, Australia
e-mail: Johannah.fahey@monash.edu

H. Prosser
e-mail: howard.prosser@monash.edu

M. Shaw
e-mail: matthew.shaw@monash.edu

J. Fahey et al. (eds.), *In the Realm of the Senses,* Cultural Studies and Transdisciplinarity in Education, DOI 10.1007/978-981-287-350-7_1

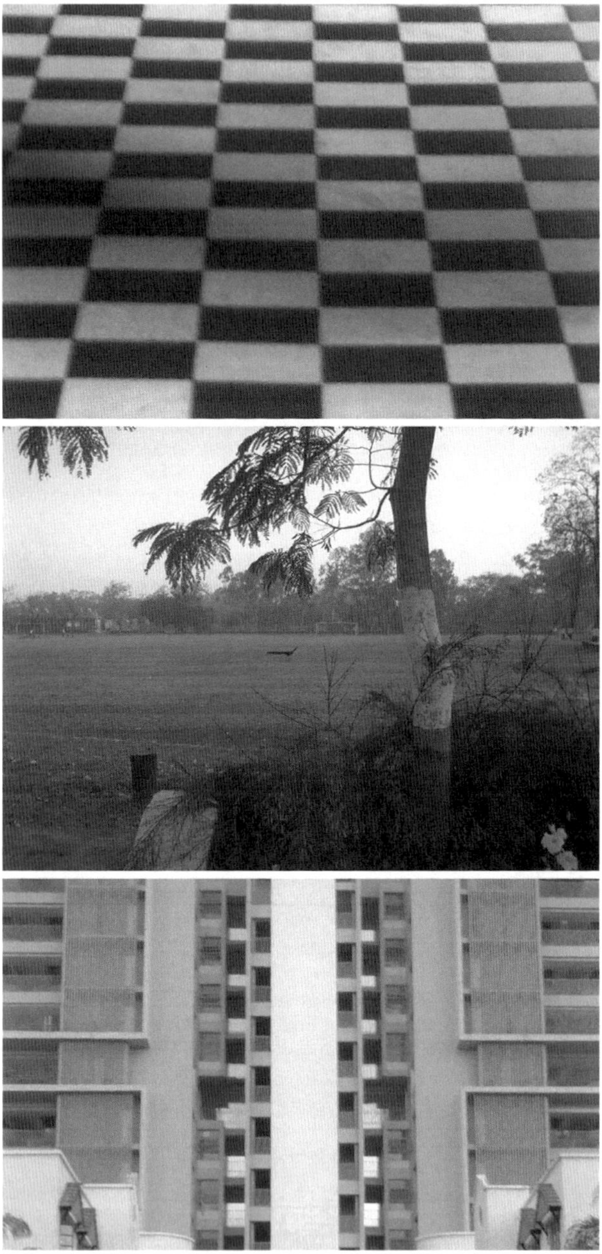

Fig. 1 'Cultural Patterns' of Highbury Hall (England), Ripon College (India) and Straits School (Singapore)

for the sons of the British East India Company's employees and the boys of local leaders in the new British colony of Singapore, with its carefully manicured greenery contrasting with condominiums, terrace houses and an industrial estate.

Elite Schools[2] The 'elite schools' we discuss in this book are all based on the British public school model.[3] In addition to the school in England itself, the others are located in former colonies, such as India, Singapore, Australia, Barbados, Cyprus, Hong Kong and South Africa. Additionally, one of the schools is located in Argentina, which was a part of the informal empire.[4] Our work seeks to build on understandings of elite schools by examining a range of schools that, while established by the British or during their period of ascendency in world affairs, are from a range of different countries with very different experiences of colonialism and post-colonialism.

There is, of course, no standard definition of what constitutes an 'elite school'. We understand them to be those which enjoy the greatest reputation and standing within their society due in part to their high academic standards and their provision of a well-resourced (from fees and benefactions), well-rounded education, which invariably leads students to tertiary studies at the world's elite universities,[5] or the leading universities in their nation. They also have proud and celebrated (usually self-celebrated) histories and notable alumni that they mobilize to separate them from other schools (Fig. 2).

A vast range of co-curricular activities are integral to the well-rounded education these elite schools offer, these are particularly in the arts and sports but also increasingly in global youth leadership programs, such as the Model United Nations, and community service programs (Kenway and Fahey 2013). A high percentage of the students that attend elite schools come from wealthy families, including families who are influential figures in the social, cultural, political or business worlds (Hartmann 2007). Research conducted in the UK, USA and Australia suggests that, while these schools serve these dominant social groups, they can also provide a means of social mobility for students who are admitted to the school but who are not from such privileged backgrounds as their classmates (Jones and Kavanagh 2003).

---

[2] The contributors to this book are all members of a research team studying *Elite Independent Schools in Globalising Circumstances* (2010-2015 ARC DP1093778) led by Professor Jane Kenway. The project is a multi-sited global ethnography that is interested in the ways in which elite schools deal with changing social conditions as a result of increasing globalization.

[3] These are long-established and exclusive schools in England that charge considerable fees. For example, Winchester traces its history back to 1382, Eton to 1440, Rugby 1567 and Harrow 1572. These are just four of the 'Clarendon Commission' schools that are viewed as the prototypical British 'public schools'. They initially started as charity schools but by the nineteenth century chiefly educated the sons of political, economic and social elites and adopted a disciplined and athletic model of education. This public school ethos (witnessed largely in specific codes of behaviour, speech, and appearance) although inculcated in so few students is thought historically to have had influence over both the British nations and the British Empire. A form of this public school ethos still exists in contemporary times and continues to be linked to a particular sort of influence and social standing.

[4] The British did not control the political or administrative mechanisms of the state of Argentina, but did have a considerable social and economic presence because of their role in the state's trade and infrastructure development.

[5] In rankings of universities by a number of sources, such as QS World University Rankings; the Times Higher Education World University Rankings; Shanghai Jiaotong University; and Academic Ranking of World Universities (ARWU), Oxford, Cambridge and the Ivy League universities in the United States invariably are considered elite universities.

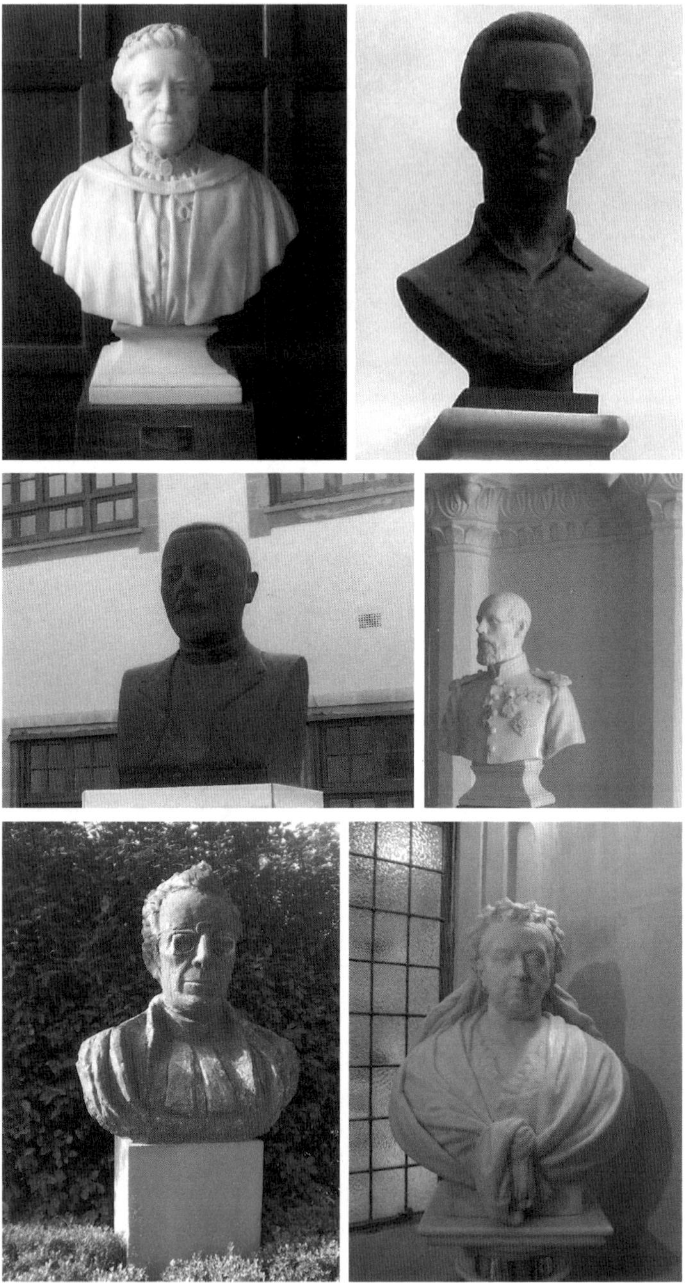

Fig. 2 Eminent figures from our elite schools in England, Cyprus, India and Argentina

In England, many of the most prestigious schools were established long before the Empire reached its zenith during the Victorian and Edwardian eras but it was during the second half of the nineteenth century that these schools flourished. Their growth was precipitated by the industrial revolution and the expansion of British influence throughout the world, which resulted in a newly wealthy class of businessmen. These men wanted social standing to go with their recently earned wealth and initially sending their boys and subsequently their girls to these schools was one means of trying to achieve this social mobility. The students at these schools were the children of gentlemen, noblemen, and clergymen who possessed the social status the newly wealthy desired and wished to acquire (Thompson 1992). This served the social aspirations amongst the newly wealthy since it educated their children into the same culture as those of established wealth and standing.[6]

The expansion of the British Empire during the second half of the nineteenth century meant that many of the men, who were in the imperial service as part of the administration or as military officers in the colonies, had attended these schools (Mangan 2000). This was also the case with those who were not a formal part of the British hierarchy in the colonies but who had, perhaps, gone to do missionary work or further their own or their family's business interests. Schools were established in these locations by some of these former public school students, especially members of the clergy, and they modeled them on the ones they had attended in the UK. These schools then became prominent in colonial settlements—which usually lacked much in the way of secondary education—and drew their students from members of the British community (or at least from those members that could not afford to send their children back to the UK for their schooling) and from amongst members of the non-British communities in the colony. But, it should be said, that this was not always the case. Other schools that we now see as linked to these British public schools do so retrospectively in a context of contemporary globalization: affiliation with such schools is now an identifiable signifier of excellence. Some catered to local elites, like Maharajas in India, or to more humble colonial functionaries, as in Cyprus or Argentina.

Nowadays, although the height of the Empire's power is now in the distant past, the reputations of these schools have been maintained by their adjustments to changing social conditions and thus their continuing to appeal to high-status social groupings (Mills 1956/2000; Kliebard 1995; Bourdieu1984; Bourdieu and Passeron 1977/2000). Their alumni continue to be found in highly important and influential positions in the business, professional or political worlds. For example, Eton College's reputation for producing a significantly higher number of British Prime Ministers than any other school stands as testament to this (Rubenstein 1993). In the past, elite schools educated the British aristocracy and catered to families with wealth, but even today, while the students who attend the elite schools under discussion may not necessarily be from wealthy backgrounds, as a result of their schooling these students are invariably provided with academic and social advantage.

[6] Our understanding of 'culture' throughout is informed by Arjun Appadurai's suggestion that it has 'great potential for giving people some understanding of the world they are in, of where they fit, and of where they are going to go'. He also maintains that culture is 'not something extra outside economy, but crucial to the economy' (2010 online).

Social Aesthetics

It is one thing to conjure up images of these schools in one's head and indeed present photographs of them, it is another thing entirely to actually immerse oneself as a researcher in these environments. Despite the fact that all these schools are very different, and even though they all have distinct histories, when one is in these spaces although expressly nuanced a commonality emerges: a palpable sense of privilege. Of course, the experience of moving through these spaces is not determined by the environment and our interactions within that environment alone, we also come into these places burdened with our own perceptions of and expectations about elite schools informed by a theoretical relationship to them and by our own biographies. The ways in which we perceive these schools and then make sense of them 'is guided by cultural, intellectual and personal interests' (MacDougall 2006, p. 2). As a means to navigate our embodied encounters within these schools, and extend these subjective experiences into a larger theorizing of social relations that considers the ways in which privilege works within these elite schools around the world, we mobilize the notion of 'social aesthetics'.[7]

David MacDougall, a visual anthropologist, develops this concept from his own fieldwork in an elite Indian boarding school during the late 1990s. The series of five films that emerged from his research—beginning with *The Doon School Chronicles* (2000, 2001a, 2001b, 2003, 2004)—offer insight into the daily lives of staff and students in the school.[8] The films' composition also highlights the school's cultural traits with an eye to its everyday accoutrements—moving images of student interactions are placed alongside still shots of their uniforms or school flags. For MacDougall the combined effect of such factors influence the interpretations of a social setting. This gives rise to the idea of social aesthetics as 'a range of culturally patterned sensory experiences' (MacDougall 2006, p. 94) that are often overlooked in ethnographic research. Social aesthetics affects people's actions just like the other factors—economic, political, and religious—that e/merge in examined communities (MacDougall 1999). MacDougall's work in the Doon School demonstrates social aesthetics at play, usually unwittingly, through the cultivation of specific experiences within the school grounds—the effects of which are felt by the students, staff, and visitors (ethnographer included) as well as the viewers of the film.

MacDougall has argued that European Enlightenment understandings of aesthetics—value judgments of art or objects—should be avoided when thinking about social aesthetics (1999). Instead a broader definition of aesthetics as simply the perception of things, which is much closer to the original meaning of the term *aisthetikos*, offers far richer interpretive possibilities. Aesthetics are thus liberated from a banal association with preference and emerges as an individual's perception of

[7] Elite schools are not the only places in which social aesthetics can be read. All social situations have their own aesthetics that are sensorily experienced. Yet elite schools are useful sites to highlight this concept because they have clear visual codes that are synonymous with conventions of social privilege.

[8] MacDougall has also written extensively about the school and its 'social aesthetics'.

anything and experience of the things within their sensory field. No longer is it simply a matter of taste; rather aesthetic appreciation is more experiential and random than an engagement with a work of art. In other words, the aesthetic realm is all that is experienced by the individual in a particular location. Certain preconceptions are brought into this experience and hence there is a pattern to the individual's response.

Just what creates these patterns is difficult to determine. Part of the reason is likely a human predisposition to make the unfamiliar familiar. This leads to codification and meaning making. But even before this point there is an experiential or phenomenological response that is part of the sensory experience of our environment. This experience is ultimately an aesthetic encounter with the material world in an unsignified way. As a result, the experiential nature of the material aesthetic precedes our rational codification or interpretation of it, if only momentarily.

But soon the experience becomes interpreted through our own subjectivity. The social nature of this perception becomes crucial. Aesthetic experiences are composed of perceiving a variety of culturally defined meanings. These meanings have their own histories as well as current social conventions that allow them to be understood in the present. In MacDougall's work, the social aspect of aesthetics thus refers to how a society or group, such as the school community, derives certain understandings through encounters with the fabric of their daily lives. A school community, for example, understands 'a particular structure of sense impressions, social relations, and ways of behaving physically' that determine their perception of the world they inhabit (MacDougall 1999, p. 16).

This approach potentially offers a new way of thinking about social dynamics within this context. MacDougall sees his formulation of sensory experiences as adding to the way historians and ethnographers see the world as well as represent it. Methods that address the senses, he suggests, offer an opportunity to move beyond 'knowledge as meaning' and 'embrace knowledge as being' (MacDougall 2006, p. 6). For MacDougall film is central to such reconsideration. Through film, the visual and auditory data can be collected that engage the senses. Likewise, film provides a means of exploring and interpreting social experience. This can then lead to new forms of knowledge not envisioned by text-based media and requiring a language that represents the multidimensionality of the subject (MacDougall 1999).

Our engagement with this concept begins with the understanding that social aesthetics relates to the 'creation of an aesthetic space or sensory structure' (MacDougall 2006, p. 105) The idea that in any given social space the senses construct the social space and make it meaningful and that without them the space per se would not be fully comprehensible ('the senses' and 'sensory structure' will be discussed in more detail below). We believe that social aesthetics is a rich interpretative notion for understanding the dynamics of privilege in elite schools and the ways in which elite schools around the world sustain their privileged status. While MacDougall's understanding of social aesthetics is an appropriate place for us to start, it is also our intention to develop his ideas and thus move beyond them. This is done in two interrelated ways: one, which we begin with, is methodological; the other is theoretical.

Social Aesthetics (Methodological Perspective)

MacDougall has written about social aesthetics and also represented this notion filmically in his video documentaries depicting the 'small "constructed"' (MacDougall 1999, p. 4) Doon School community. When writing about social aesthetics he says that he recognizes 'that the school exist[s] within (and was interdependent with) a complex national, as well as global, economy and culture' (MacDougall 1999, p. 4), and yet he does not tend to elaborate this point. He also deliberately avoids portraying this broader complexity in his films, concentrating instead on the school and contributing to the construction of it as 'a world in miniature' (MacDougall 1999, p. 4), as a place that provides students with a life determined entirely within the school walls. MacDougall is primarily conveying the students' experiences as they are felt inside the school community rather than showing how the school produces social elites—the latter of which is done in the work of Sanjay Srivastava (1998).

While MacDougall focuses on one school in a single country, we focus on multiple schools across multiple countries. Our extended scope of analysis allows us to view social aesthetics within each site as well as in relation to the others. Other scholars who have written about elite schools in the US (Khan 2012; Gaztambide-Fernández 2009; Howard 2008), England (Walford 1986; Maxwell and Aggleton 2013), and Australia (Connell et al. 1982) tend to view society as nationally bounded (Dale and Robertson 2007). Studying multiple schools in multiple countries that share a common status as elite schools means that we are able to consider a complex of 'small societies' across the globe and the ways in which they sustain each other, but also contemplate the ways in which these small societies are interdependent with a world beyond the school gates: with their localities, their regions, and with contemporary globalization (Kenway and Fahey 2009). We too are interested in these elite schools as a microcosm of life, but we are also attentive to their relationship to macro effects in the world at large (Burawoy et al. 2000). Therefore while elite schools do indeed have their own local context, although these surroundings are by their very nature exclusive they are nonetheless never truly distinct from, and are always in interaction with, broader global processes.

Photo as Metaphor How then do we grasp this complex sensory and aesthetic environment? One way to begin is to picture, if you will, the researcher in this environment taking up the mantle of ethnographer in the field. When thinking about the ethnographer in the field one quintessential visual that comes to mind is that of a Malinowskian figure: the white man seemingly integrated with the black tribesmen in the environs of a remote village in Melanesia (Fig. 3[9])

Why does this image, above all others, come to mind? Perhaps it resonates as it is seen to be the epitome of ethnographic convention and it speaks to the tradi-

[9] This is a photographic file from the Wikimedia Commons. This file is in the public domain. It has been identified as being free of known restrictions under copyright law, including all related and neighboring rights.).

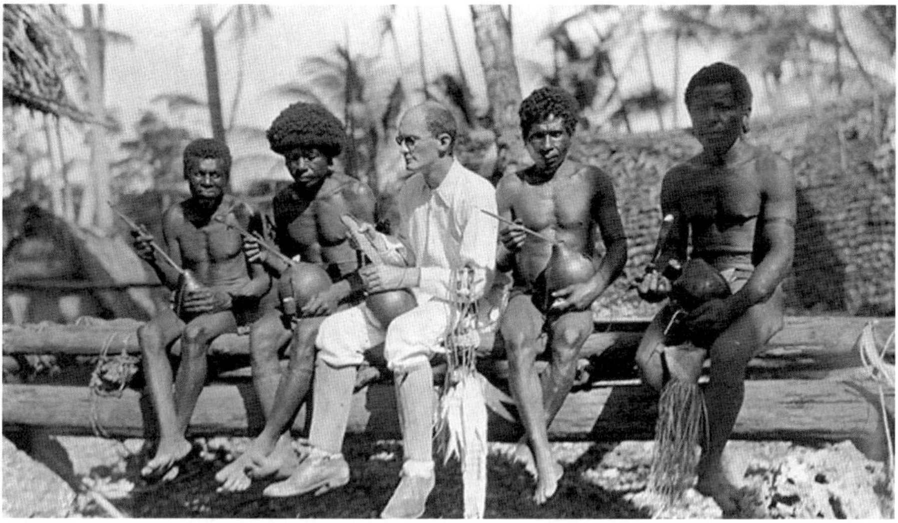

Fig. 3 Malinowski with 'natives'. (Trobriand Islands, 1918)

tional notion that 'the power of ethnographic fieldwork is … held to derive from long-term immersion and thick description' (Epstein et al. 2013, p. 470). Obviously, when seeking to understand the complexities of an unfamiliar sensory and aesthetic environment the idea that we immerse ourselves in these surroundings over a long period of time is a compelling one. Indeed, this is precisely what Prosser and Shaw did, in the solid 6 months they spent undertaking fieldwork in Argentina and Cyprus respectively. And yet, for the most part, with regard to our team's fieldwork this was not our modus operandi. Imagine instead relatively brief visits to the field for the duration of 3 or 4 weeks each over a period of 3 years.

Without the luxury of time, capturing the ephemeral everydayness of the field is not accomplished easily. As an ethnographer in the field our work still involves the daily practice of immersing ourselves in our research environment. However knowing that the time is limited does add 'an intensity and urgency to the fieldwork that, perhaps, sharpen the acuity of [not just] the ethnographic gaze' (Epstein et al. 2013, p. 470) but the other sense experiences as well. Within such an environment our sense experiences become finely tuned and hypervigilant; having said that, once we have left the field such experiences can rapidly fade. To retain these experiences we write field notes on a daily basis, and once out of the field reading back over them does much to jog the memory. But it is the photographs that we have taken in the field that best act as visual prompts depicting particular instances and taking us back in time to what Cartier-Bresson (1952), the French photographer and 'father' of modern photojournalism, calls the 'decisive moment', to places and faces that stare back at us from the recent and sometimes distant past (Fig. 4).

The art critic John Berger suggests that the image 'is a site which has been recreated or reproduced … which has been detached from the place and time in which it first made its appearance' (1972, p. 9). This is an important suggestion for us as

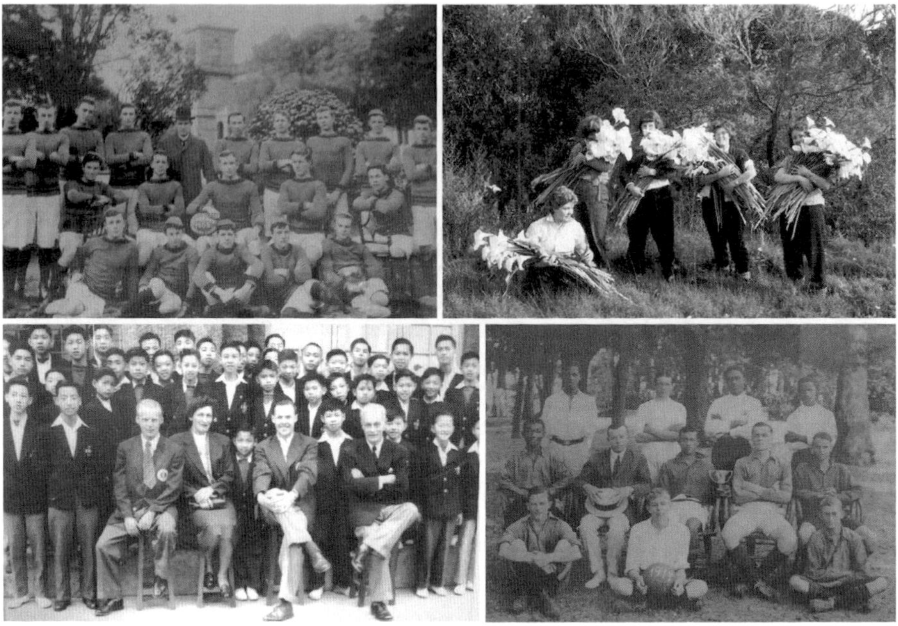

Fig. 4 Archival photos from Founders (Australia, 1900s), Greystone (South Africa, 1980s), Cathedral College, (Hong Kong, 1950s) and Old Cloisters (Barbados, 1900s)

we are interested in social aesthetics in terms of social relations and social context. Therefore rendering the place and time from which the photographic image has been detached is of particular significance. In analogue photography the photographer isolates their shot by peering through the viewfinder and cutting off the scene that lies beyond the frame. In digital photography the viewfinder has been enlarged. It is, therefore, no longer the case that in pressing one's eye flush against the sight the world is reduced to a mere rectangle flooded with light. Nowadays the camera is held at a slight distance and whilst the shot is seen within the screen the world beyond also remains in full sight. These different modes of taking photographs are perhaps a useful way to think about and develop Berger's point.

On the one hand, as the photographic image is a single de-contextualized shot it has in some ways been detached from its original place and time, as Berger states. This process of disconnection provides a fitting metaphor for understanding our approach to this collection of writing and images. In the same way in which a photographer captures an image by isolating a particular part of the landscape within the viewfinder, while the wider social aesthetics environment of elite schools is our focus, we nonetheless use the photograph as the lens through which we enter this broader theoretical terrain. At the same time, we problematize the ways in which photographs are severed from the context in which they were taken by considering below the relationship between our textual chapters and our visual essays.

On the other hand, somewhat paradoxically, although the photographic image is a single de-contextualized shot it nonetheless becomes a proxy for the time and place in which it was taken. The photograph can be thought of here as a part that represents the whole. Within the photograph's borders the time and place of its taking have a residual presence that contributes to the very meaning of the image. According to Berger, 'a photograph, whilst recording what has been seen, always and by its nature refers to what is not seen. It isolates, preserves and presents a moment taken from a continuum' (2001, p. 217). That continuum can be thought of as a continuum of meaning, a process of trying to make sense of what we see, and trying to determine how what we see relates to what we don't see.

MacDougall astutely captures the relationship between taking images and making meaning, when he says 'images reflect thought, and they may lead to thought, but they are much more than thought' (2006, p. 1). He characterizes this thought process not in terms of language (as is customary), but rather in terms of 'ideas, emotions, sensory responses, and the pictures of our imagination' (MacDougall 2006, p. 2). When conducting ethnographic work the daily practice of seeing is very much about our being in the world, it is about bringing a 'feeling of being into our seeing' (MacDougall 2006, p. 1). What this means is that our ways of seeing and the ways in which we derive meaning from what we have seen cannot be divorced from who we are: our emotional, sensory, and corporeal reactions as well as our ideological or political proclivities are shaped by social aesthetics.

The moment in which the ethnographer makes a decision that the event before them is significant and deemed worthy of a photo, is of equal importance to the moment when a photograph is taken. In other words, when trying to determine more about the time and place in which the photo was shot we must also seek to know more about the person who took the photograph. In this regard, the ethnographer's way of seeing cannot be separated from the person that has created the image. An understanding of social aesthetics, therefore, entails understanding ways of seeing as 'physical [and decisive] encounters' (MacDougall 2006, p. 1) as the ethnographer makes certain choices in the instant that they capture a shot. As Berger states (2001, p. 216):

> If everything that existed were continually being photographed, every photograph would become meaningless. A photograph celebrates neither the event itself nor the faculty of sight in itself. A photograph is already a message about the event it records. The urgency of this message is not entirely dependent on the urgency of the event but neither can it be entirely independent from it. At its simplest the message, decoded, means: I have decided that seeing this is worth recording.

In the process of taking a photograph we have therefore made an aesthetic judgment with regard to something in particular that we have seen in our vast visual field. Szarkowski, the photographer, curator and critic, talks about the process of taking a photograph, saying: 'the central act of photography, the act of choosing and eliminating, forces a concentration on the picture edge—the line that separates in from out' (2007, p. 9). In broader terms too specific aesthetic judgments have been made. For instance, there is the moment when the school (or rather its representatives) decided which visual imagery it would display on the basis of how it wanted the school to be perceived; there is the moment within the school when we, as ethnographers, took the original picture; there is the moment when we decide which photos best illustrated our research endeavors; and there is also the moment when we, as editors, decided which photographs to include within the pages of this book to illustrate our thoughts. Here we are fully aware of MacDougall's warning that 'meaning, when we force it on things, can also blind us, causing us to see only what we expect to see or distracting us from seeing very much at all' (2006, p. 1).

By drawing attention to these moments of decision we recognize that our selection of images is based on a process of inclusion and exclusion. We also acknowledge that such a process undoubtedly affects ideas of representation and perception, and that there are certain limitations on the images' ability in this book to capture the social aesthetics that we talk about entirely—not least of all because our representations of our sensory experiences have been reduced to mere visuals and text. We also admit that even in the field our ability to record our environment was curtailed by limitations placed on us by the schools, but also by other kinds of limitations. In this respect, La Grange points out that in contemporary times 'photographs themselves have become so widespread, and their subject matter so all-encompassing that is has changed both what we think is worth seeing and, in terms of ethics, what we think we have a right to see' (2005, p. 30). In terms of the schools, precisely because of ethical concerns, many of them requested that we did not take photographs of their students. And yet, while this is clearly an ethical issue about what the school thought we had a right to photograph and what we did not, perhaps this ability to choose who sees what can also be thought of as a certain kind of privilege, the following anecdote provides some illumination with regard to this idea.

In order to get a sense of where our research school fitted in relation to the broader educational landscape and a wider social context, and as a way to interact with the larger community, we visited a village school just outside the gates of the elite school we were researching in a bustling industrial Indian city. The village school was a marked contrast to the beautified surrounds, and all that they imply in terms of privilege, of Ripon College. It was located on a main road where the stream of motorbikes and auto rickshaws was never ending, and where there were no towering walls or trees (unlike those at Ripon College) to protect the school's students from the traffic or the dust that arose in its wake. The school catered largely to impoverished children, some of whom attended the school simply to be provided with what would be their only meal for the day. When standing in the school grounds the students gathered around one researcher and she started taking photographs, largely as a means to communicate in the absence of a shared language. She would take a shot and then show it to the students in the photograph much to their delight. But in reflecting upon her visit to the village school, the researcher did wonder if taking photos of the students at this school was at all appropriate, asking herself, 'if I was a parent of one of these children would I approve of a complete stranger taking photographs of my children?' Of course, this situation was made more complex by the fact that she was not only a stranger, but also a foreigner. Here then the ethics of assuming a tourist gaze also come into effect. In the act of taking a photograph certain power dynamics exist and negotiating these dynamics is clearly one indication that one is ethically engaged in the situation. MacDougall says that 'our consciousness

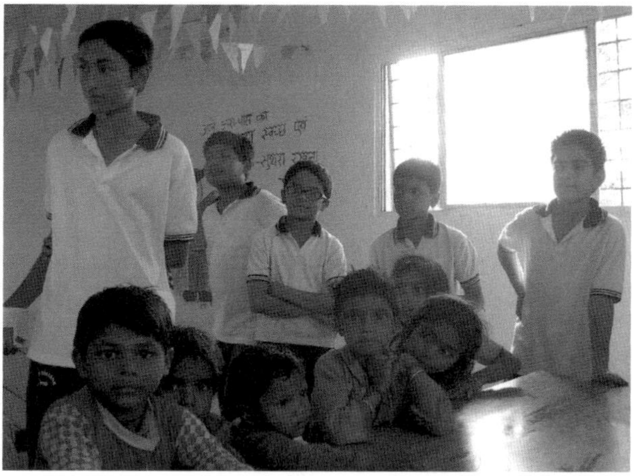

Fig. 5 A way of seeing Ripon College students and children from a nearby village (India, 2013)

of our own being is not primarily an image, it is a feeling'[10]. In this instance, feeling uncomfortable led to ethical questions that serve to remind us that we must always be aware of the broader social aesthetics that determine a social context, not just in which a photograph is being taken, but also in which research is being conducted (2006, p. 1; Fig. 5).[11]

Elite Schools as Deliberately Ahistorical Elite schools aim to exude an image of perpetual steadiness. This image makes them seem assured, reliable, and confident. It also promotes a school community ideal that MacDougall characterizes as 'inward-looking, ahistorical, conservative and self-perpetuating' (1999, p. 17). But this, as MacDougall also makes clear, is a myth that undermines the dynamism of these school communities. While the idealized 'world' of the Doon School appears unchanging in his films, his intention was the opposite: they also alert us to the ideological nature of this affect.[12] Certainly the idea that elite schools, which arguably

[10] We acknowledge that social aesthetics does have affective and emotive dimensions. While we do not enter into a detailed theoretical engagement with affect and emotion here we do explore these themes in the sensory vignettes throughout the book.

[11] Thinking about aesthetics and ethics calls to mind Ranciere's (2006) work on the relationship between art and politics. He has an aesthetic conceptualization of politics (the notion that aesthetic acts should be thought of as a confluence of sensory experiences that create new forms of political subjectivity) and a political conceptualization of aesthetics (the idea that the political state of society at a particular time determines the political meaning of art) However, while these are both interesting concepts, as his definition of politics—where he distinguishes between 'politics proper'(*le politique*) and the police order (*la police*)—is a complex one, referring to his work in more depth here would obscure rather than clarify our concerns.

[12] It is important to note that by representing the school in this way MacDougall perpetuates the insularity of the school, and that there is a particular ideology (i.e. the durability of exclusivity) at work in the persistence of this ideal. In this respect, what actually becomes 'self-perpetuating' is the ideology itself and this virtuous circle necessarily informs the elite status attributed to such schools. In his essay, 'The Doon School Reconsidered', MacDougall remarked that 'the school culture was by no means static' (p. 129).

represent the ideal school community, are enduring insular environments, exclusive islands unto themselves, is a convincing one. The continuity of these schools as high-status communities is created in part through their dependence on the fortunes of their school community and their former students. Nostalgia is a powerful force, but it only goes so far in assisting social reproduction.

Moreover while it is possible to frame the establishment of the schools we will be discussing in terms of a definitive historical moment (i.e. British colonialism), it would be wrong to assume that the effects of British colonialism were experienced in the same way in each country and therefore in each school (Hall 1996). Here a paradox emerges. Although each school may have a unique 'stamp' (MacDougall 1999, p. 96) that leaves a lifetime impression upon its students, this 'distinctive material signature' is a commonality that unites all elite schools. The notion that elite schools leave a stamp suggests that they are 'sensory structures' that bear a material signature of privilege, social aesthetics, which signifies itself differently within larger social aesthetics. In other words, this stamp is not particular to the Doon School, but rather is particular to elite schools, despite the fact that they all strive to be exceptional. And yet, at the same time, they *are* all exceptional as the ways in which they experience the lingering effects or the aftermath of British colonialism cannot be understood in the same way in these sites. Rather the influence of postcolonialism is experienced differently in each place and there are thus important nuances within each of these post-colonial educative environments.

Furthermore, while elite schools undoubtedly honor their histories and traditions, in contemporary global times they are also engaged in strategies of innovation as a means to reinvent themselves and thus remain relevant. Therefore, while in some respects they are conservative, many of the schools in our study aspire to being seen as liberal, progressive environments. These schools draw upon influences from both the community within which they are located and are subject to the forces of contemporary globalization that influence educational practices. Indeed, the schools we discuss in the coming chapters are acutely aware of their place as educational leaders in their own locality and the need to keep up-to-date with both curricular and pedagogical trends in order to maintain their reputations.

MacDougall initially wrote about social aesthetics at the end of the twentieth century. Nowadays, having already lived beyond the first decade of the twenty-first century, we are writing in a different historical period where significant changes have taken place. We do not seek to frame MacDougall's 'little worlds'—'of family and school' hierarchically in terms of 'a larger world that they encountered in the streets, during their travels, and on television' (MacDougall 1999, p. 17). Rather, we conceive and configure the 'little worlds' on the ground in different countries in different elite schools in contemporary globalizing circumstances in terms of a co-constitutive relationship where each is defined horizontally, in relation to the other (Popkewitz and Rizvi 2010).

One of the major differences in contemporary times is that we more readily communicate in images. The digital technological revolution has facilitated this process by making every citizen with access to a computer able to create their own visual sensibility—from doctoring personal photographs to producing, and uploading, quotidian footage for all to see on picture sharing social networks such as Facebook, Instagram, Tumblr or Flickr. Today's global suffusion of advertising culture—the beguiling propaganda of contemporary capitalism—has also contributed to the creation of image-centric societies around the world. All of this serves a larger scheme of social relations once linked to spectacle (Debord 1995) and consumerism but now, with the move from a 'read only' to a 'read-write' culture (Lessing 2009), intertwined with consumption *and* production. Therefore, although we acknowledge the limitations of only using photographs to depict the wider realm of social aesthetics, given the predominance of the visual in today's world there is also some justification in privileging the visual (in the form of photographs) in this collection (Howells and Negreiros 2012).

Visual Essays It is entirely possible for a solitary photograph to represent a certain moment and for the viewer of this photograph to interpret the significance of this moment. In this interpretive instance a broader context that exists beyond the photograph's frame is nonetheless implied as a kind of absent presence that contributes to the ways in which the viewer makes sense of this single image.

In choosing to include visual essays in this book we are not only gesturing to the power of the visual in constituting social aesthetics, we are also constructing a context for each photograph with other photographs, thus making these photographs meaningful in another way. The function of the visual essays is to provide 'an ongoing text of photographs' whereby 'context [serves to replace] the photograph in time—not its own original time for that is impossible—but in narrated time' (Berger 2001, p. 292). As one photo follows another a visual narrative unfolds like a film slowly spooling frame by frame across the page.

Here we not only theorize the visual, but also allow the visual to speak for itself, so to speak. The effect of viewing photos is different to reading essays or interviews. 'Appearance *is* knowledge, of a kind. Showing becomes a way of saying the unsayable' (MacDougall 2006, p. 5; Fig. 6). Were we to have merely written

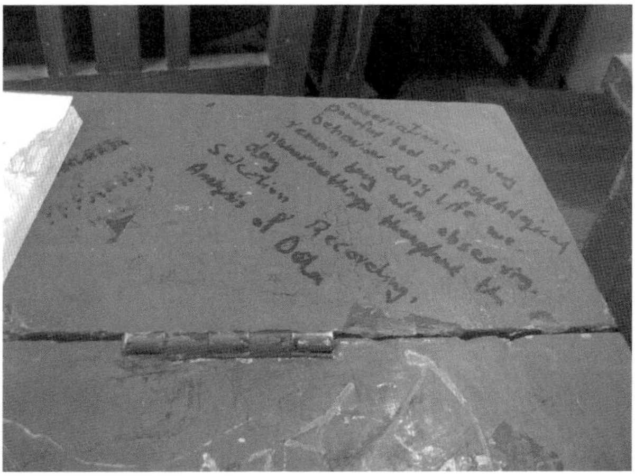

Fig. 6 'Text of photographs', school desk (Ripon College, 2012)

about social aesthetics, our interpretation would implicitly devalue the potential for the image—the photo, in this case—to offer critical insight. The visual essays put the 'photograph back into the context of … social experience [and] social memory' (Berger 2001, p. 292), and situates our portrayals of social aesthetics in a wider socio-historical context. These images are sequenced to create a visual resonance and relationship between each photograph where one photo refers back to the photo that precedes it or follows it in order to generate meaning. Through the visual essays we do not seek to return each decisive photographic moment back to the continuum from which it was taken. Rather, there is a deliberate effort to consciously juxtapose one photograph beside another as a means to explicitly depict certain power relations and portray a particular political sensibility. In presenting a montage of images from our fieldwork we contend that the power of social aesthetics is contained precisely in the positioning of various constitutive parts.

The visual essays cannot, of course, offer much beyond impressions of the various schools and their surroundings. As Douglas Harper suggests, photos are a series of windows unfolding aspects of culture, but the view is incomplete (Harper 2013, p. 14). Elite schools create such an aesthetic context for themselves, wittingly and unwittingly, via the use of images in their own yearbooks, advertising, websites, or foyers. Many of the schools differed in the way that eliteness was on display: these displays must be viewed within the totality of the social context. As is obvious from some of the pictures, some of the schools do not replicate the imagined ideal of cultivated gardens or cloistral passages. This upsets any popular images of elite schools by revealing their global variance. Our purpose is not to merely duplicate the sense of privilege the schools promote. Rather we are suggesting that an essay of images can critically illuminate and abstractly represent the prevailing social conditions that allow elite schools to dominate. Put another way, we are pointing to the fact that photographs capture social contexts that may serve as representations of the dynamics of privilege in action.

Moreover, there are limits to still photography as a visual representation of the social aesthetics versus a film or video. Photos capture moments as they took place but lack the dynamism of film. MacDougall's medium and argument overlap in this instance because the dynamics of the social aesthetics are best experienced through video footage. Such footage is able to express the living experiences of individuals in a more subjective way.

We offer a broader context in the visual essays, as well as with photos throughout the book, by mobilizing historical traces that constitute a social experience not limited to the schools' grounds. The result, we hope, is a sense of social aesthetics that cannot be simply expressed in the textual snapshots of other chapters. Indeed, the visual essays should offer just as much a sense of what constitutes social aesthetics as this theoretical introduction. The visual essays are an abstract intervention in the social aesthetics of elite schooling around the globe.

Making Sense of Class Making (Theoretical Perspective)

When reflecting on his experiences at the Doon School, MacDougall refers to the school as 'a specially constructed kind of society with its own distinct boundaries' (Kildea and MacDougall 2012, p. 55) he also observes the 'aesthetics of power' at play in the ritualized disciplining of the students' bodies (Kildea and MacDougall 2012, p. 57). However while MacDougall speaks about privilege in relation to power and exclusivity he doesn't speak about privilege in relation to social class specifically. For us the relationship between privilege and class is a pivotal theoretical intervention that is crucial to understanding the ways in which social aesthetics function in the elite schools we discuss. In this context, we examine how class is connected to the dynamics of privilege, and how privilege is related to power. Therefore our understanding of politics, and the politics of power, herein is articulated to our understandings of privilege and our concern with the ways in which class interests are reinforced through a particular social aesthetic and a certain sensory structure built on the nexus between privilege, power and class in these schools.

Class and Social Aesthetics Class is difficult to talk about largely because it is hard to know precisely what we mean when we are talking about class. Another reason that class is difficult to discuss is that so much has been said about it in the past. Perhaps the most instructive place to start then is to define the ways in which class is conceptualized. Rather than survey the intricacies of scholarly debates, the positions can be simply, and perhaps simplistically, described in the opposition between the dominant Marxist and Weberian positions. Of course, the divide is not set fast, and there are limits to the dogmatic appropriation of both: a commitment to either ahistorical or stratified class systems, for example. Yet enough has been written to suggest that when class is understood through social relations it is fruitful to combine these positions (Aronowitz 2003). Drawing predominantly on sociologist Erik Olin Wright's conflation of Marxist and Weberian approaches to class, we maintain that class is understood as a form of social division that is determined by economic and cultural exchanges (2008). This approach is in keeping with the ongoing discussion about how best to read class distinction in light of important contributions to social theory. Rather than subscribing to an either/or position—which sees the economic or the cultural as the most important factor in determining class—we believe culture and economics inform each other. This eschews a hierarchy of knowledge and instead adopts what Wright calls a 'pragmatist realism' (2009, p. 101). Economic *and* cultural attributes shape people's opportunities and choices in a market economy and thus determine their social class. Consequently, class influences the way people interpret the world not by placing them in a specific category but positioning them in ongoing social processes. Such processes are thus made up of different interpretations of material conditions based on sensory experiences of particular contexts.

Class and Social Relations Social relations affect peoples' material interests. It is not the case that people live in separate spheres of material life isolated from one another. But rather, that the material conditions of peoples' lives are lived in relation to other peoples' spheres of material existence. It is through the articulation of these relations, which serve to link different class locations, that we come to understand class in relational terms. Economically, we conceptualize class as social relations that connect people to capital and to each other through the exchanges of these commodities. That is, it is market exchange that determines social relations, or as Weber (1978, p. 927–928) maintains, "'class situation' is, in this sense, ultimately, 'market situation'". Or, alternatively, according to Marx: 'it is not the consciousness of men that determines their existence, but their social existence that determines their consciousness' (Marx 1987 [1859], p. 263). Culturally, we recognize that the materiality underpinning these relations occurs and is interpreted differently in various contexts, even in spite of globalizing circumstances. As such class characterizes itself as a process within different, if related, contexts. Stuart Hall's work provides a knowing guide in this matter precisely because he underscores the importance of the economic interwoven with the social and cultural. For this reason, gender and race remain as important as the economic in determining privilege. Such an intersection of factors means that the specifics of class politics in various locations are always distinct. In colonial settings, as Hall points out, the classical Marxist analysis of capitalism's installation overlooks local peculiarities influencing its entrenchment—as in the South African social formation where, for example, the 'economic relations are the necessary, but not the sufficient conditions of racial structure' (Hall 1980, p. 310). Therefore, race and ethnicity clearly add important dimensions to our understanding of social aesthetics. We are particularly interested in the intersection of social aesthetics and the historical specificity of the contexts and environments in which race and ethnicity become meaningful. This includes understanding the tensions that are generated by the uneven direction and development of race and ethnicity in different times and places, and the ways in which social aesthetics contributes to social differentiation, the social divisions and contradictions that arise around race and ethnicity in this historically-shaped terrain. It is precisely these disparities and disjunctures that emerge around the inter-relationship of class, race and ethnicity, both within and across particular countries that we explore in more detail in later chapters.

Social Relations and Social Context If we posit that a theory of class is a theory of social relations then we must also recognize that these social relations necessarily operate within a social context. Which is to say, that class is not an objective social category, rather it is influenced by a certain set of circumstances. There are different ways in which to think about social context, however rather than presenting an exhaustive list, we will simply provide some pertinent illustrations.

For example, social context can be thought of as being constituted over time and in particular places.[13] That is, social context is informed historically in terms of the period of time in which people live, and geographically in relation to the country that they live. Both these attributes contribute to the social context of social relations, and thus understandings of class. In contemporary times, one of the key ways

[13] In this way we seek to avoid essentializing 'the' social context as a generalized phenomenon.

of framing this social context is in terms of the contemporary capitalist economy. And yet, the on-the-ground effects of this global economy will necessarily be distinct in different countries. In terms of the latter, the culture in which people live and the institutions with which they interact within such cultures will also contribute to the construction of a social context. The state too, which can be understood as 'the sphere of direct enforcible [sic] social relationships (as against the indirect relationships of the market)' (Connell 1977, p. 5) is integral to establishing a social context.

Of course, when talking about 'social context' we are not just thinking about the immediate milieu or spatial environment. Although these are determining conditions in relation to class they are not the defining limits of a given social context. Social context can also be experience according to one's gender or race; families, neighborhoods, and networks between individuals and organizations can also be determining factors that provide the social scaffolding for social relations.

Educational Social Contexts The culture that people are educated in, the educational institutions that they attend (if they attend any at all), and the educational resources that this affords them, can also all be thought of as contributing to a social context. Given the focus of this book, education as social infrastructure is of particular interest to us. More specifically, educational settings are excellent starting points for considerations of social aesthetics because of their foundational role in the experiences of individuals and their broader function as re/producers and reconfigurers of social class.

It is our contention that the social context associated with elite schooling has a distinctive sensory dimension. To put it another way, social aesthetics can be read in class terms through the way that the social context is experienced in elite schools. MacDougall gestures towards this idea when he talks about a unification of "the sensory with the 'cultural' landscape" (2006, p. 2). He further states that he is interested in 'societies themselves as complex sensory and aesthetic environments [and]... the importance of these settings of human life as they exist in experiential terms' (MacDougall 2006, p. 2). For us, societies are indeed complex sensory and aesthetic environments that are experienced through social relations that are ultimately class bound. We are interested in the ways that elite educational institutions, as a particular kind of exclusive society, contribute to the understandings of social relations and class theory.

Sensory Vignettes

Further ethnographic texture is given to the elite schools in this book via the vignettes that appear throughout the texts. These short texts describe some of the researchers' experiences of their locales via four senses: hearing, seeing, touching, and tasting/smelling. The purpose behind such illustrations is to offer an experiential interpretation of social aesthetics at different schools. Our purpose is to show how the textual can represent more than a theoretical analysis of the social aesthetics and get closer to representing, ironically, its 'unsignified' nature. The power of ethnographic research and writing often lies in the personal experiences of the ethnographer. These experiences can be evoked within short narrative structures that capture moments or processes in ways that photographs cannot. So, the vignettes, in a manner similar to the visual essays, reveal the social aesthetics of elite schools as not being bound by their fences or gates: a clamorous bus ride to an elite school in Barbados; the visual dissonance of arriving at an elite schools' Cyprus whose grounds don't quite fit the envisaged expectations; the feeling of being included in an elite Argentine school or the sensation of being beckoned by the aesthetics of eating in an elite South African school. These descriptions offer ways of representing social aesthetics in an auto-ethnographic fashion and perhaps offer a glimpse of how it may be described further in the future by those in such spaces.

Patterned Sensory Experiences Snapshot

For MacDougall (1999, p. 7), social aesthetics consists of many elements 'not so much in a list of ingredients as a complex, whose interrelations as a totality (as in gastronomy) are as important as their individual effects'. The methodological and theoretical perspectives we have outlined above come together in the chapters that follow and guide us through the intricacies of this 'complex'. In these pages the authors detail the ways in which the sensory structure of elite schools, composed here of cultural, corporeal, spatial, and temporal scaffolding, gives them a specific characteristic. All of these factors contribute to the sense of being in these schools and how such being—through the effects of social aesthetics—translates into belonging, estrangement or ambivalence. Such inclusion or exclusion is then directly linked to the way that social power manifests in these privileged educational settings and beyond.

Each chapter can be thought of as a 'snapshot' of social aesthetics' constituent parts. The concept of a snapshot offers a partial and thus imperfect representation of the social aesthetics of which we speak. Our textual snapshots are impressions, representations, or abstractions of social aesthetics' sum; they are not equal to it. Each chapter is the ethnographers' impression of social aesthetics at particular elite schools with a link to specific socio-theoretical interventions of the past few decades. Hence, MacDougall's social aesthetics theory is situated alongside the likes of Lefebvre, Berger, Bourdieu, Appadurai, and Benjamin.

Yet, like the vignettes and photos, each chapter offers something of a critical intervention into the production of elite schools' social aesthetics while simultaneously contributing to the reader's imaginary impression of actually being in an elite school. Although the chapters isolate each sensory experience—be it cultural, temporal, spatial or corporeal—from the total social aesthetics landscape, there is nonetheless an interrelation between each. Further, the textual aspect of the book has been arranged in a way that incorporates different ways of 'writing' about the social aesthetics. The vignettes are one example of this, but so too are more traditional scholarly essays, and a combined textual/visual essay. These chapters are outlined below.

Space and Social Aesthetics The spatial is especially important because the location and grounds of elite schools are always central to their identity. Externally, an elite school's location is always related to affluence and influence: either positioned close to political and economic power centers or in desirable parts of the city or nation. Internally, the ability of these schools to imbue social privilege makes their location representative of power too. The school's security systems go a long way to confirming this position, but so too do the range of facilities that are being secured. This is especially the case in the elite schools located in the Global South—South Africa and Argentina—discussed by Kenway and Prosser. In these settings spatial distinctions pronounce racial and class divisions. The image of hyper-secure homes and private neighborhoods in these nations is common; elite schools are also vigilantly protected. But it is not just security that comes to mind when talking of space. Privilege is obvious in the size of the schools grounds relative to that offered students in non-elite schools. This translates into privilege in material terms through the school's offering greater room and resources than elsewhere. In South Africa and Argentina, where urban space is often at a premium, the way the elite schools in our study have been designed, built, and used reveal a history of entitlement as well as ongoing social influence. Such supremacy only exists in relation to the contrast of its surrounds. This chapter, following the lead of Lefebrve (1991), elaborates on the changing spatial practices used in these elite schools, especially since the establishment of liberal democracy in both Argentina and South Africa in the last few decades. By focusing on the spatial aspect of social aesthetics there is scope to understand how elite schools not only position themselves as outside broader society, and how this position is also crucial to the dynamics of the city or town in which they are located.

Semiotics of Social Aesthetics Social aesthetics lends itself to articulating semiotic methods and theories. In his chapter, Koh draws out some of these themes in his consideration of semiotics, social aesthetics, and ethnography in regard to Straits School—an elite school in Singapore. Koh's approach is to measure the usefulness of social aesthetics to what he sees as a necessary turn to semiotics in ethnographic writing. Straits School is saturated with signs with their own affects, which invited interpretation. In coming to terms with these signs Koh suggests that a theory of 'semiotic ecology' is appropriate and can complement the idea of social aesthetics. Koh reads the way that twenty-first century artifacts—school-branded bottles of mineral water and large printed banners designed to inspire—are coded with presumptions about privileged presents and futures. These sit alongside images from the past to create sediments of meaning that assist with the formation of elite identities as well as offering rich veins of potential data for ethnographers.

Cultivating Students' Bodies Bodies 'inhabit social spaces but also create them' (MacDougall 2006, p. 127). More specifically, students' bodies are materialized and normalized in certain ways in elite schools, but students' bodies are also utilized to form the sensory environment that is particular to these elite schools. Focusing on two elite schools, in Cyprus and Barbados, Fahey and Shaw begin this chapter by examining the physical body in relation to sport and the political and ideological boundaries that exist between the Greek Cypriot and Turkish Cypriot students.

Boundaries created by particular social aesthetics dominate the real and imagined landscape on the island and the school is one of the few sites that makes an active attempt to cross them. It is, however, also a site in which cultural, social and historical forces interact to ensure their preservation. This chapter considers sport as one means of breaking through boundaries but also as a site where conflicting ideologies meet. The use of the body in this space, or its withdrawal from it, is a means by which students attempt to maintain control of their own ideology and identity. Attention then turns to the ways in which poetics and politics contribute to the representation of particular kinds of racialized bodies. The aesthetic and political dimensions of real or imagined bodies are linked to bodies as subjects and the articulation of subjects, the state, politics and economy. In the Barbadian school, the content of the students' artwork is intrinsically linked to the promotion of an 'ideal Caribbean' identity, as a means to leverage regional affiliation and as a way to compete on a global stage. While the corporeal is singled out here as our point of focus, the body is also thought of in relation to our other sensory categories and as a complex and contested product of entwined material, social, cultural and historical forms (Featherstone et al. 1991; Turner 1996).

Postcolonial Social Aesthetics Given that social aesthetics of elite-ness can vary from place to place, McCarthy et al consider how post-colonial social aesthetics may be theorized and measure MacDougall's theory against other major contemporary thinkers. Paying attention to the sensory structure of elite schooling takes on a heightened significance in the post-colonial school setting, where a school in a former colony, an elite school based on the 'metropolitan paradigm' in Barbados, literally wrestles with the future. McCarthy et al outline how this school uses a vocabulary of tradition as it seeks to better prepare its students for the transforming circumstances of both tertiary education and occupational choices generated in the global context. This chapter suggests that this elite school, situated as it is in the post-colonial setting, is a sensory site of curation and consecration in which colonial condensations abound along with markers of indigenizing and globalizing registers of change and transformation. This is a vibrantly hybrid and contradictory cultural context. The photos used throughout the chapter reveal how images and artifacts of the past are used in the present as part of the student's identity—as post-colonial performers with global futures. These aesthetic markers are inlaid in the rich imagery of the everyday rituals of school life, the artifacts and emblems of school identity, the architectural forms of school buildings, the curricular texts and materials used in the classroom. Along with this are the vigorously imaginative universes of real and vicarious action verbalized by students in their interviews with researchers. This chapter shows that the field of these social aesthetics are densely overlaid with the markers of the historical past etched in objects and practices that are profoundly indigenizing, nationalizing and globalizing.

Making Sense of Social Aesthetics Entering the gates of an elite school elicits a variety of feelings based on the individual's relationship to such institutions and the power they represent. Some of these gates, like those at Ripon College in India, are laden with meaning. In this chapter, Rizvi reflects on his own experiences of fieldwork at this elite school. These experiences are positioned in relation to his theoretical reflections on social aesthetics. Rizvi's thoughts are particularly important since his own approach to an Indian school differs somewhat from MacDougall's take on the Doon School. For Rizvi, theorizing social aesthetics is complicated by the different 'aesthetics' experienced. He also considers how the social is defined within social aesthetics suggesting that it incorporates relational aspects of the national and the global. A large part of this relationality is the way that the school defines itself against what is outside its gates. This has a significant impact on what happens at the school—what is taught and what is expected of the students once they leave.

Conclusion

This book is a transdisciplinary collection that speaks across the disciplines, and uses numerous theoretical sources, and empirical data to develop and problematize MacDougall's seminal work on social aesthetics. In doing so it brings together critical discussions of new empirical research and allies them to established theory to develop new theoretical knowledge around the concept of social aesthetics. It scrutinizes the aesthetic nature of social relations in elite schools in terms of a broader context, including the context of globalization. It departs from conventional studies of elite schools that merely focus on their social purposes and concentrates instead on the manner in which sensory experiences are part of the class-work of elite schools—how they are involved in social class configurations, processes and relationships in intersecting colonial, post-colonial/national and transnational terms.

The shape of the book is also deliberately unconventional. We have arranged the text with a substantive introduction to present social aesthetics as worthy of critical scrutiny with a mind to its mobilization and appropriation in the ethnography of elite schooling. We also believe it deserves even wider consideration in other scholarly fields. To do justice to the theory and its possible methodology, we have used photographs throughout the book to capture moments of social aesthetics in process. These photographs acknowledge and complement MacDougall's own medium—film and video—as well as present ethnographic research in ways that do not rely on the written word.

The visual essays, in particular, betray the power of the visual in our interpretation of privilege, especially in relational terms. Unlike MacDougall's *Doon School Chronicles*, we show the life outside of the gates of the schools that is integral to the social privilege that is in motion within them. Readers can form their own interpretations of these images, some of which are repeated elsewhere in the book. The written sections also work to eschew the usual formalities of edited collections by constituting a blend of genres—the scholarly essay and a text-cum-visual essay. The cumulative effect is designed to capture social aesthetics at its instantaneous moment of experience as well as when it begins to be interpreted through a theoretical lens.

Social aesthetics must therefore be seen in both theoretical and methodological terms. It seeks to capture a convergence of sensory factors that contribute to an experience of social relations in specific locations and across time. As a concept it need not be confined to ethnography. Although ethnography is an approach that is certainly well suited to considering social aesthetics precisely because it can capture—through text, film, recording or other means—aesthetics not as preference but as sensual experience. Theoretically, a number of existing social theories can be employed to provide a better rendering of social aesthetics. The means of analysis can be appropriated from elsewhere. Semiotics is a case in point; although the visual should not be the only signifier under consideration: where visual semiotics may assist with our reading of images, other sensory semiotics would also be needed. Methodologically, there are lots of challenges since the idea of social aesthetics seeks to capture a holistic experience that is fleeting and read in different ways. But our point is that certain locations, like elite schools, repeat the experience, albeit in slightly altering ways, for those attending the school each year and thus create a pattern that can be read by those living and visiting the environment—like an ethnographer—for an extended period.

Consequently, sensory responses that may at first seem insignificant become extremely significant precisely because they signify the feelings exuded by the social privilege of elite schooling. Considering these elite schools with a mind to their social aesthetics is ultimately what this book seeks to achieve. MacDougall's work offers an important starting point for this endeavor. The authors in the collection offer suggestions on how to develop this work in light of contemporary theory as well as developments in contemporary ethnographic methods. We hope that this dialogue offers the next step in considering and using of social aesthetics to understand the social dynamics of privilege, and its opposite, in globalizing circumstances.

References

Appadurai, A. (2010). Arjun Appadurai on culture and its possible impact. Forum d'Avignon. http://vimeo.com/23264628. Accessed 20 June 2013.

Aronowitz, S. (2003). *How class works: Power and social movements*. New Haven: Yale University Press.

Berger, J. (1972). *Ways of seeing*. Harmondsworth: Penguin.

Berger, J. (2001). Understanding a photograph. In G. Dyer (Ed.), *Selected essays* (pp. 215–246). London: Bloomsbury Publishing.

Bourdieu, P. (1984). *Distinction: A social critique of the judgement of taste*. Cambridge: Harvard University Press.

Bourdieu, P., & Passeron, J. C. (1977/2000). *Reproduction in education, society and culture*. London: Sage.

Burawoy, M., Blum, J. A., George, S., Gille, Z., & Thayer, M. (2000). *Global ethnography: forces, connections and imaginations in a postmodern world*. Berkeley: University of California Press.

Cartier-Bresson, H. (1952). *The decisive moment*. New York: Simon & Schuster.

Connell, R. W. (1977). *Ruling class, ruling culture*. Cambridge: Cambridge University Press.

Connell, R. W., Ashenden, D., Kessler S., & Dowsett G. (1982). *Making the difference: Schools, families and social division*. Sydney: Allen & Unwin.

Dale, R., & Robertson, S. (2007). Beyond methodological 'Isms' in comparative education in an era of globalisation. In R. Cowen & A. M. Kazamias (Eds.), *Handbook on comparative education* (pp. 1113–1128). Netherlands: Springer.

Debord, G. (1995). *The Society of the Spectacle,* translated by Donald Nicholson- Smith, New York: Zone Books

Epstein, D., Fahey, J., & Kenway, J. (2013). Multi-sited global ethnography and travel: Gendered journeys in three registers. *International Journal of Qualitative Studies in Education 26*(4), 469–487.

Featherstone, M., Hepworth, M., & Turner, B. S. (1991). *The body: Social process and cultural theory*. London: Sage.

Gaztambide-Fernández, R. A. (2009). *The best of the best: Becoming elite at an American Boarding School*. Cambridge: Harvard University Press.

Hall, S. (1980). Race, articulation and societies structured in dominance. In UNESCO (Ed.), *Sociological theories: Race and colonialism* (pp. 305–345). Paris: UNESCO.

Hall, S. (1996). When was the postcolonial? Thinking at the limit. In I. Chambers & L. Curti (Eds.), *The post-colonial question: Common skies, divided horizons* (pp. 242–260). London: Routledge.

Harper, D. (2013). *Visual sociology*. Abingdon: Routledge.

Hartmann, M. (2007). *The sociology of elites*. Abingdon: Routledge.

Howard, A. (2008). *Learning privilege: Lessons of power and identity in affluent schooling*. New York: Routledge.

Howells, R., & Negreiros, J. (2012). *Visual culture*. London: Polity.

Jones, B., & Kavanagh, D. (2003). *British politics today* (7th ed.). Manchester: Manchester University Press.

Kenway, J., & Fahey, J. (Eds.). (2009). *Globalizing the research imagination*. London: Routledge.

Kenway, J., & Fahey, J. (2013). Staying ahead of the game: Elite secondary schools' globalizing curriculum practices. *Globalisation, Societies and Education, 12*(2), 177–195.

Khan, S. R. (2012). *Privilege: The making of an adolescent elite at St Paul's School*. Princeton: Princeton University Press.

Kildea, G., & MacDougall, D. (2012). Discussion between David MacDougall and Gary Kildea about Doon School Chronicles. *Humanities Research, XVIII*(1), 55–70.

Kliebard, H. (1995). *The struggle for the American curriculum*. New York: Routledge.

La Grange, A. (2005). *Basic critical theory for photographers*. Burlington: Focal Press.

Lefebrve, H. (1991). *The production of space*. Oxford: Blackwell.

Lessing, L. (2009). *Remix: Making art and commerce thrive in the hybrid economy*. New York: Penguin Press.

MacDougall, D. (1999). Social aesthetics and the Doon School. *Visual Anthropology Review, 15*(1), 3–20.

MacDougall, D. (2000). *Doon School Chronicles*. [Film], Berkeley Media LLC.

MacDougall, D. (2001a). *With Morning Hearts*. [Film], Berkeley Media LLC.

MacDougall, D. (2001b). *Karam in Jaipur*. [Film], Berkeley Media LLC.

MacDougall, D. (2003). *The New Boys*. [Film], Berkeley Media LLC.

MacDougall, D. (2004). *The Age of Reason*. [Film], Berkeley Media LLC.

MacDougall, D. (2006). *The corporeal image: Film, ethnography and the senses*. Princeton: Princeton University Press.

Mangan, J. (2000). *Athleticism in the Victorian and Edwardian public school: The emergence and consolidation of an educational ideology*. Abingdon: Routledge.

Marx, K. [1859] (1970). Preface. In M. Dobb (Eds., Introduction), A contribution to the critique of the political economy (pp. 19–23). New York: International Publishers.

Maxwell, C., & Aggleton, P. (2013). Becoming accomplished: Concerted cultivation among privately educated young women. *Pedagogy, Culture and Society, 21*(1), 75–93.

Mills, C. W. (1956/2000). *The power elite*. New York: Oxford University Press.

Popkewitz, T., & Rizvi, F. (2010). Globalization and the study of education: An introduction. In T. Popkewitz & F. Rizvi (Eds.), *Globalization and the study of education* (pp. 7–28). Malden: NSSE.

Ranciere, J. (2006). *The politics of aesthetics*. London: Bloomsbury

Rubenstein, W. D. (1993). *Capitalism, culture and decline in Britain, 1750–1990*. London: Routledge.
Srivastava, S. (1998). *Constructing post-colonial India: National character and the Doon School*. London: Routledge.
Szarkowski, J. (2007). *The photographer's eye*. New York: The Museum of Modern Art.
Thompson, P. (1992). *The Edwardians: The remaking of British society* (2nd ed.). London: Routledge.
Turner, B. S. (1996). *The body and society*. London: Sage.
Walford, G. (1986). Ruling-class classification and framing. *British Educational Research Journal, 12*(2), 183–195.
Weber, M. (1922/1978). In G. Roth & C. Wittich (Eds.), Economy and society: An outline interpretative sociology (Vol. 1). Berkeley: University of California Press. (Part-I, Chapters 1, 2).
Wright, E. O. (2008). The continuing importance of class analysis. In L. Weis (Ed.), *The way class works: Readings on school, family and the economy* (pp. 25–43). New York: Routledge.
Wright, E. O. (2009). Understanding class: Towards an integrated analytical approach. *New Left Review, 60*, 101–116.

Johannah Fahey is Senior Research Fellow in the Faculty of Education at Monash University, Australia. Her research interests are located in the areas of education and global studies, and are informed by her expertise in cultural studies. She has a national and international reputation in the areas of intersectionality (gender, race and class), and cultural globalization and mobilities. She is the co-editor of *Globalizing the Research Imagination* (Routledge 2009); and co-author/author of *Haunting the Knowledge Economy* (Routledge 2006) and *David Noonan: Before and Now* (Thames and Hudson 2004). She has also published in many eminent international journals and edited books. She is the leading Research Fellow on the international team conducting the research project called *Elite independent schools in globalising circumstances: a multi-sited global ethnography*.

Howard Prosser researches and teaches in the Faculty of Education, Monash University, Australia. He has taught history in Australian secondary schools and universities. His research interests include Social Theory, History of Ideas, and Ethnography. Most recently he has been working on a study of political culture at an elite school in Argentina.

Matthew Shaw is a PhD candidate in the Education Faculty at Monash University, Melbourne. His interests lie in history including the history of sport as well as the place of sport in schools and society. His dissertation looks at the role sport has in a divided society and the way it is used to reinforce or break down boundaries.

Vignette: The Fullness of Taste

Jane Kenway

What does privilege taste like? Is there a link between the palate and the palette? Is taste tinted? Tainted?

High on the slopes of the mountain in Cape Town, is Greystone with its 'award-winning, architect-designed' pre-preparatory school for girls from 3 to 6 years of age. No classroom has more than 24 students. This light filled, spacious school also has a 'child-friendly, landscaped garden environment'[1]. Playground equipment is crafted to look like Africa's wild animals. Multi-coloured frescos, murals, learning equipment and beanbags add charm. Even the toilets have a designer touch; multi-shaded, carefully matched small tiles, quirky angles, artfully arranged basins. White spots adorn the girls' red aprons worn to protect their pale blue peter-pan collared uniforms. The mothers too adore colour. Their dazzlingly joyful Mad-Hatter's Tea Party tables are festooned with flowers, balloons, candles and draped beads. One table has fine china with delicate pastel floral patterns and quaint candelabrum. For their ballet performances the girls wear pale pink, but elsewhere vivid pink is their colour. In the passageway their school bags, lunch boxes and water bottles are predominantly pink and red. In the playground a pink and blue cubby house awaits. And at the Mad-Hatter's Tea Party there are copious servings of heart-shaped biscuits, iced in pink and red, and decorated with little silver balls and swirls of purple and glitter.

To me, this school tastes pink. Sweet.

On a flat and dusty street of downtown Cape Town, is a government school attended by black children from the townships. Facilities are well kept but basic, school 'décor' is restricted to the front lobby. Assemblies are held outside on the hard earth, under a rare tree. There are roughly 60 students in each crowded

[1] These quotations are from the school's website.

J. Kenway (✉)
Monash University, Melbourne, Australia
e-mail: jane.kenway@monash.edu

J. Fahey et al. (eds.), *In the Realm of the Senses,* Cultural Studies and Transdisciplinarity in Education, DOI 10.1007/978-981-287-350-7_2

classroom—all eager. The school provides students a lunch of mieliepap. Made from mielie-meal this porridge/polenta is a staple food of South Africa's many poor. Inexpensive, eaten with vegetables, it is their everyday food. In a small, hot, smoky shed at the school two elderly, tired, women stand for the morning stirring and watching over two big vats in which the mieliepap is boiled. High in carbohydrates and protein and quite low in fat, it is filling and reasonably nutritious. In its more up-market version, in the fashionable cafes on the hillside near Greystone, mieliepap is accompanied by meat, vegetables or a savoury sauce, or, in homes that can afford meat, it is served as a side dish at *braais* (barbecues). To these hungry children, however, it is dispensed unaccompanied, but liberally. It is filling. On its own, dull-white and stodgy, it is humble and unappealing fare.

To me this school tastes tenacious. Gritty.

There are two main types of taste. First there is taste-bud taste, tongue taste—sweet, sour, salty, savoury (umami) and bitter. Secondly there is life-style taste. This may be associated with those perceived as distinguished, cultured, or stylish, those with breeding, those who can make refined judgments. They have impeccable taste, not simply, the more modest, good taste. On the other hand there are those seen to lack taste, to have no taste, poor or bad taste; those who lack judgment, refinement, civility, who are uncultured. In both instances taste is associated with things, appearances and behavior.

Lifestyle taste is not always straightforward. Good taste, too visibly or carefully cultivated, can be a bad sign; a sign of anxious social striving, of not having quite arrived. Further, while the distinguished can have momentary lapses and behave in ways considered to be in poor taste, the undistinguished cannot, it seems, have lapses of impeccable taste. As this suggests, lifestyle taste is ordered hierarchically.

In addition though, taste-bud taste and lifestyle taste cannot be readily separated. The thing of food, its aesthetics and the act of eating are, together, implicated in hierarchicies of taste. The food one eats, its look, where one eats, how and even why are often socially, as well as ethnically, coded. The class codes, for example, of fast food and fine dining, processed foods and whole foods are readily readable. Scarcity boosts price.

Of course these class codes are also scripted. 'Taste classifies and classifies the classifier' (Bourdieu 1984, p. 6). This well-known aphorism reminds us that taste always has its cultural intermediaries—those who assess, ascribe and guide values and value. They can be regarded as the arbiters of what, in many ways, is culturally arbitrary.

Taste is also tainted. Mega-corporations control much of the world's food production and distribution. They target for profit the addictive tastes of the tongue—fat, salt and sugar. Yet the poor may be stigmatised for their unhealthy food/lifestyle choices (Patel 2008). And with its links to the slave trade from Africa and to slavery on the sugar plantations of the West Indies in the eighteenth century, sugar's history leaves a bitter after-taste. There is nothing arbitrary about the link between food and poverty; it involves the tastes of necessity under-pinned by an economy where scarcity is a norm not a choice signaling superiority. Poverty does not have many tasteful food affordances.

References

Bourdieu, P. (1984). *Distinction: A social critique of the judgement of taste*. Harvard: Routledge and Kegan Paul (Trans: Richard Nice).

Patel, R. (2008). *Stuffed and starved: Markets, power and the hidden battle for the World Food System*. New York: Portobello Books Ltd and Melville House Publishing.

Jane Kenway is Australian Research Council Professorial Fellow, Professor of Global Education Studies at Monash University, Australia, and an elected Fellow of the Academy of Social Sciences, Australia. Her research expertise is in socio-cultural studies of education in the context of wider social and cultural change. Her more recent jointly edited books are *Asia as Method in Education Studies: A Defiant Research Imagination,* (Routledge 2015) and *Globalising the Research Imagination* (Routledge 2009). Her more recent jointly written books are *Masculinity Beyond the Metropolis* (Palgrave 2006) and *Haunting the Knowledge Economy* (Routledge 2006). She has published numerous book chapters and journal articles. She leads the international team conducting the research project called *Elite independent schools in globalising circumstances: a multi-sited global ethnography*.

Distinguished Spaces: Elite Schools as Cartographers of Privilege

Jane Kenway and Howard Prosser

If a space is produced, if there is a productive process, then we are dealing with *history* (Lefebrve 1991, p. 46; original emphasis).

Introduction

Elite schools are aestheticized spaces. Their grounds are cultivated by a team of workers with an approach as assiduous as the manner in which the teachers attend to their students. This manipulation of space—buildings and gardens—seeks to fit with a range of ideas about how these schools should look, often with cues taken from colonial metropoleis and local vernaculars. Such imaginaries materialize a sense of beauty that resonates with the rationality of the education being conducted within the schools' boundaries.

But they are no more socially aestheticized than any other parts of the cities they inhabit. Here our use of social aesthetics seeks to look beyond the expected surrounds of such schools and examines how they fit into specific social relations, particularly race and class, that have changed significantly in the last few decades. Our focus is on two elite independent schools: Greystone in South Africa and the Caledonian School in Argentina.[1] There is a number of similarities between the situations in South Africa and Argentina in the last few decades. The most striking is the transition to democracy since the 1980s. To be sure, many nations have

[1] Howard Prosser conducted the fieldwork in Argentina; Jane Kenway and Debbie Epstein did so in South Africa.

J. Kenway (✉) · H. Prosser
Monash University, Melbourne, Australia
e-mail: jane.kenway@monash.edu

H. Prosser
Monash University, Melbourne, Australia
e-mail: howard.prosser@monash.edu

J. Fahey et al. (eds.), *In the Realm of the Senses*, Cultural Studies and Transdisciplinarity in Education, DOI 10.1007/978-981-287-350-7_3

undergone this shift during this period. But there are two aspects that are interesting for our study. First, as part of this shift there has been the attempt to create a new sense of collective identity in both nations: South Africa has confronted of race while Argentina has seen some realignment of class. Sometimes this process has managed to further reinforce social differences. Second, these nations have moved from a state system of security to one that was quickly privatized for those who could afford it. Securitization is a global phenomenon, certainly. But both South Africa and Argentina involve striking instances of such security concerns that, at a moment of expressed civic intentions, have brought forth a guarded reaction on the part of the wealthy.

Top-notch schools in Argentina and South Africa use their space to respond to these changes in similar ways. As bastions of privilege under periods of authoritarian rule, although not directly complicit with these regimes, they served the groups that thrived under these political conditions. With the arrival of more liberal political leadership in their respective republics, these schools have had to accommodate, or at least think about accommodating, the social other—black and poor—while at the same time, defending themselves from perceived threats to their security. As a result, the ways in which the schools define, and defend, their spaces have changed with differing degrees of accommodating an open society that is, paradoxically, increasingly privatized.

In both instances, this is a historical process that has clear spatial manifestations. These can be described in relation to the ways that privileges become enclosed by and within the schools, but also within and between larger contexts. The social aesthetic of an elite school is defined, like most things, by what it is not. There is thus a spatial relationship between what is considered *of* and not *of* the school. In his work on the Doon School, an all-boys boarding school in India, David MacDougall presented a more hermetic view of the school's social aesthetics. The imagery in his films is striking for the presentation of patterns with meaning. These patterns—flags, uniforms, sculptures, gardens—appear to derive their significance from the school culture itself.[2]

We are keen to build on the idea of social aesthetics but to consider it as more broadly and dialectically determined. We focus on space. Instead of just presenting how the schools look or even function we want to reveal how they work within cultural contexts with specific histories. The spatial significance of our elite schools is dependent on how the schools sit within their cities as well as how the space is utilized. In other words, the patterns of meaning in the school are reliant on the social relations that permeate the schools' fences and walls.

To help us flesh out our contention the work of French sociologist Henri Lefebrve is instructive. His thought helps us to comprehend how these schools and their clientele use space. We say instructive because his esoteric Marxism is compelling, but not easily explained. Still, what he calls a 'spatial triad' is perhaps the best way

[2] That is not to say that MacDougall was unaware of the external influences on this internal culture of the school. His writings on the school and other fieldwork certainly prove he was. Rather, we are suggesting that the films' focus remained within the school itself (MacDougall 1999).

to understand the human creation of urban space as the culmination of a range of factors—design, culture, history, and use. In what follows, we will briefly outline the triad and then provide some examples as to how his interpretations can illuminate our schools' social aesthetics.

'Spatial Triad'

Lefebrve's 1974 text *The Production of Space* (1991), it should be pointed out, was a political intervention rather than a textbook on applied urban theory. His stated aim was to 'detonate' Western theoretical preconceptions about city space by bringing attention to the interaction between ideas and the material and social world (Lefebrve 1991, p. 24). He was keen to show how city space was actively 'reduced' through the social processes that occur within its physical limits. A city is not a passive thing in itself, or a space consisting of 'things' (Lefebrve 1991, p. 37); rather a city is produced and reproduced through the ways it functions in time. In other words, the social interactions define the space while, at the same time, the space defines the social interactions. This chiasmus may not be the clearest explanation; even Lefebrve himself conceded that there was a certain tautology to his thinking. He put it another way: '*(Social) space is (social) product*' (Lefebrve 1991, p. 26; original emphasis).

To explicate this production process he pointed to three elements: a description of how urban spaces are *conceived, lived and perceived*. The intricacies of this theory are difficult to explain here and we won't even try.[3] Placed together these three elements—conceived, lived, perceived—reveal how a city (or indeed any spatiality) functions. First is the rational, technocratic way that a city is designed. Second is the fashion in which these designed spaces are built and then used in a functional system. And third, where radical potential resides, and is usually defeated, is the way that a city is symbolically interpreted by those who use it or think it—philosophers, artists, activists, citizens (Lefebrve 1991).

These triple determinations aren't to be separated, and Lefebrve was clear there are three entangled modalities to his schema. We might add that their social aesthetics are also entangled; or, to put it differently, that their entanglement constitutes social aesthetics. Just as MacDougall sees social aesthetics as patterns in the daily lives of those in the Doon School, so too does Lefebrve consider the overall ongoing effect of the planning, workings, and happenings of a city. The design and function have more clearly defined patterns than the unruly nature of the everyday. But it is everyday life within the spaces—the living and perceiving—that are influenced by

[3] Lefebrve identified three elements in the use of urban space: Spatial Practices, Representations of Space, and Spaces of Representation. These are a little confusing, so it's preferable, in this forum, to use adjectival definitions that Lefebrve endowed them with: Conceived Space, Lived Space, and Perceived Space. For an excellent clarifying interpretation see Rob Shields, Lefebrve, Love and Struggle: Spatial Dialectics (1999).

the built environment—the conceived—which is itself always in flux. In short, the spatial variable in social aesthetics triangulates related variables. The result is what MacDougall, in terms not dissimilar to Lefebrve's own terms, sees as a 'complex, whose interrelations as a totality (as in gastronomy) are as important as their individual effects' (MacDougall 1999).

We suggest that a consideration of the social aesthetics of the spatial triad assists in exposing the way that elite schools have reinforced their position of power in two post-authoritarian societies. By reframing the threats to their personal and economic security, in terms acceptable to the new civil societies, the schools and the social elites they serve reassert a privileged position in the urban space. In other words, liberal democracy's revival in both South Africa and Argentina has also led to the consolidation of spatial privilege for economic elites. The elite schools to which these elites send their children manifest specific social aesthetics of privilege.

Democratization and Privatization

The reinvigoration of democracy in a variety of places during the 1980s and 1990s went hand in hand with the emergence of neo-liberalism. This historical intersection meant that burgeoning liberal democracies—not just in the former Soviet sphere but in South-East Asia, Latin America, and South Africa—were keen to celebrate their citizens' political rights but without taking responsibility for them in line with the post-war model of liberal state welfare.

This free-market moment, which also coincided with globalization's latest phase, placed greater emphasis on expanding private wealth than on the provision of important social services—from amenities to education. For the latter, the outcome has been a common global scenario with its own local variations: public education systems saw their funding stalled and, as a consequence of this and other factors, private schooling, for the poor and the rich in many instances, expanded. Certainly, elite schools' stars rose even further. These schools were able to leverage their strong reputations and access to higher social classes to cater to the top echelon's demands for schooling that offered first-class results, facilities and even access to international curricula. This social and political revolution went a long way to altering the way that our schools' spaces were perceived and the social aesthetics produced.

Elite School Mobility

Two points are crucial when understanding the recent development of Argentine liberal democracy. The first is the history of Argentina since 1983. This year marked the end of a 7-year period of military rule and the restoration of democracy in the nation after more than half a century of instability and authoritarianism. After a few years coming to terms with this change, Argentina underwent a massive social and economic restructuring during the 1990s. This was the era of neo-liberal exceptionalism (or exceptionablism) under Carlos Menem that collapsed spectacularly in late 2001. The disintegration was overshadowed by the start of the 'war on terror', but it was a moment of political uncertainty and social upheaval most famous for seeing five presidents in 3 weeks and the middle-classes sliding into poverty. The recovery, however, was swift thanks largely to widespread discontent being mollified by the restoration of leftist *Peronismo* under the governments of Nestor Kirchner and Cristina Fernández de Kirchner.

Second, Buenos Aires in which Caledonian School is located, does not equal Argentina. The nation, is geographically vast and has a remarkable social diversity within this space thanks to its migrant and indigenous pasts. Buenos Aires also reflects this, but there is a greater cultural homogeneity that is due largely to the nationalizing projects of the early twentieth century in which European migrants quickly became Argentines. Such homogeneity is changing somewhat, especially because of the influx of migrants from Latin America—particularly Bolivia, Paraguay and Peru. This is sometimes called the Latin-Americanization of Argentina—a process that is spoken of in terms of the presence of poverty in the streets of Buenos Aires as well as involving an end of the supposed exceptionalism of Argentina's living standards in comparison to the rest of the continent (Fig. 1).

We outline both of these things since they highlight the determinants of the spatial dimensions of life in the city today. That is to say, the arrival of democracy has gone hand in hand with the overt presence of poverty, including impoverished migrants, and a reduced standard of living. The paradox is that for those in the up-

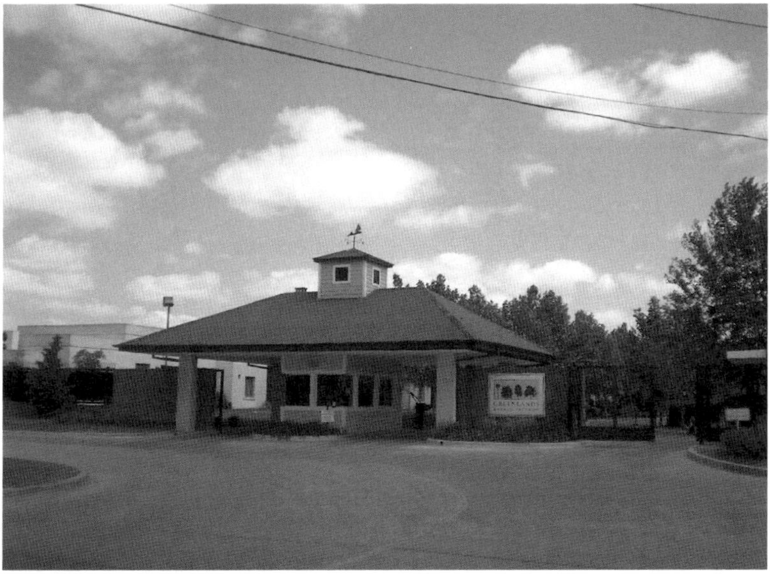

Fig. 1 Guardhouse of a closed neighborhood in Greater Buenos Aires

per echelons of society—the type of people who send their kids to the school in our study—managed to shore themselves up and even prosper during the neoliberal 1990s, and then also during its decline in the first decade of the twenty-first century. This meant that the geography of the city, which had long been divided along class lines—poor in the south, rich in the north—became more obviously defined in terms of private space and securitization. The classic example is the private neighborhood (*barrio cerrado*).

Elite private schools also embody these spatial practices. During the 1990s they became a symbol of the rich's economic success (Narodowski and Andrada 2001) and then, after 2001, of enduring prosperity: two important attributes of capitalist mentality. The conspicuous consumption of the 1990s is now frowned upon in Argentine society; but its prevalence is still obvious. In this image, for example, at an 'open day' at a prestigious 'English School' (*colegio ingles*), the car park is filled with European model cars overseen by a private security guard who's chatting with the catering firm's workers as they head back to the kitchen. The lower classes of society are only able to enter this space through their position as menial workers (Fig. 2).

At the Caledonian School, in an affluent neighborhood of the city, space has become an issue. A few years ago the school recognized the limits of its main campus space in providing for its students. It was ensconced in a suburban neighborhood without playing fields and also needed more room for classrooms and other facilities. So the decision was made to move the school to a new campus north of the city. In the next few years its current location will be sold off and a new campus,

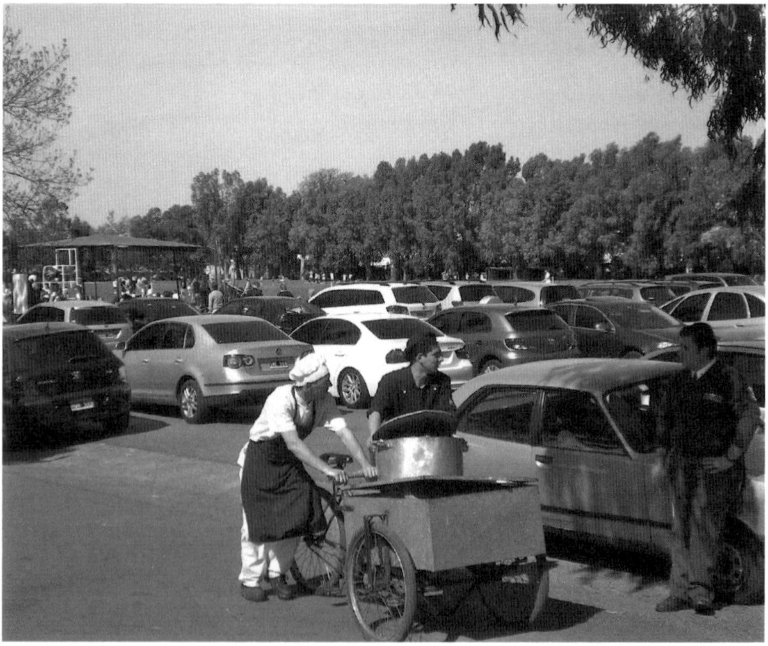

Fig. 2 Cooks and security guards converse on the grounds of an Argentine elite school during an open day

currently under construction will house a growing number of students in state of the art classrooms designed around interdisciplinarity and student-centered learning. At US$ 25 million dollars, it's an investment few other schools would be able to make.

But it is also one that is possible due to the reputation of the school being well established. Many elite schools around the world, and particularly their ex-students, find it difficult to imagine moving from their original locations due to their specific histories. Caledonian, by contrast, is much more mobile. The school's brand nods to the institution's long tradition, but innovation and excellence are stronger hallmarks. Such thinking is more like the global approach of the modern university than a primary and secondary school. This brand affords a mobility, and perhaps liquidity, that ensures the school's longevity through its affililation with a rich clientele.

There is a strong precedent for such a move. Other private schools have established campuses in to the north of Buenos Aires that are home to an increasing number of the cities affluent classes. The shift is following the future clientele. No longer are these schools' students within walking distance between home and school. Today they arrive in private buses or private cars, sometimes accompanied with security guards, from the expanding private neighborhoods to Buenos Aires's north. It's here that the new school is heading. There was a conscious choice not to place the school within one of these *barrio privados*. Many private schools opened second campuses in such neighborhoods during the 1990s. Today, there is a feeling that they are too cosseted. Caledonian wants to connect with the existing community around its new campus—such as a local secondary school that abuts the private school's site. But just what this connection will be depends on the permeability of the boundaries placed around the new Caledonian School. The gulf between the social classes that they cater for may be too great. The area is home to lower-class neighborhoods, some sections of which can be described as slums (*villas miserias*) as well as private neighborhoods. The school will stand in the middle. Even if, as one school member said to me, 'they don't want to be seen as coming in and colonizing the area,' it is hard to see how its gates and fences will not be a continuation of an exclusionary social space (Fig. 3).

During Howard's fieldwork there was, naturally, a lot of discussion about the forthcoming move. The nature of this discussion differed depending on where you were in the school. The administration were obviously all for it—they saw it as an opportunity to expand the size of the school, to offer state of the art facilities, and also revolutionize the pedagogic approach in line with computer-based, student-led philosophies. The teaching staff had more misgivings, regarding it generally as an extravagance as well as a difficulty for most of them to get to in the future. Since the majority of staff don't live in the area and instead come from the suburbs surrounding the existing campus or downtown, there may be a change to the nature of the staff as well.

This process captures the dynamics of the spatial practices that Lefebrve outlines. There is a specific design, construction and use of the areas—both existing and new—that have specific determinations along class lines. In keeping with this is changed social aesthetics. The Caledonian School, which has risen from a relatively small parochial school for Anglo-Argentines to one of the preferred choices for Argentina's economic elite, is moving from a suburban existence to one among

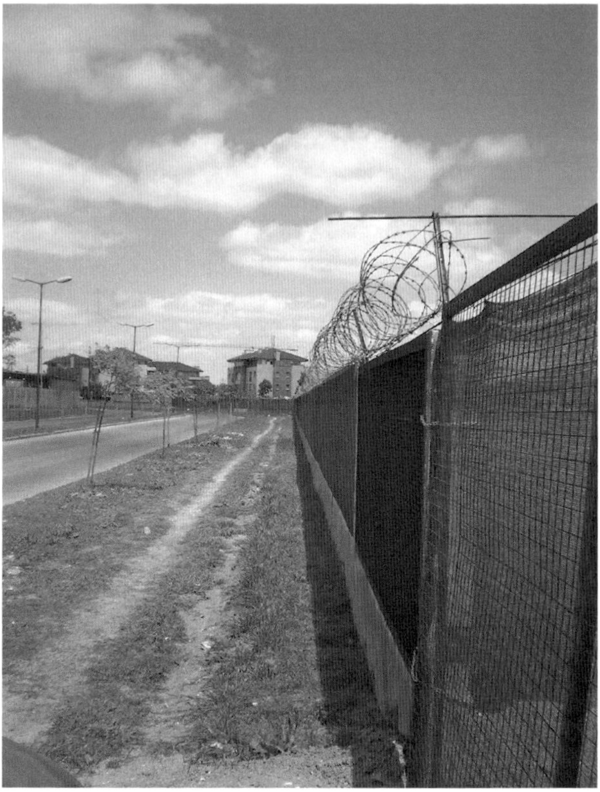

Fig. 3 The barrier of the new Caledonian campus during construction

the rich plains of the River Plate colonized by those seeking to escape the chaos of downtown. To be sure, the internal culture of the school will have some continuity; but, as with other moments in its history, the school will also enter an even more privatized space.

Spatial-Racial Practices

In South Africa, apartheid was a deliberate spatial practice. Under the National Party's minority rule, white supremacist South African society was produced through the racialization of space. White power was exercised through all aspects of Lefebvre's triad. Apartheid involved a planned, racially hierarchical, apartness, held in place, to a large extent, by the violent force of the state. Non-white people ('black' [native], 'colored' [mixed], and 'Indian') were up-rooted and shifted to out-of-the way places; they were corralled and then viciously controlled. District Six is a notorious Cape Town example of this forced movement and the rise of many poor black townships outside of the city bowl was the eventual shocking result. In the city bowl, not too far from Greystone, upmarket shopping centers and dwellings sprang up in the spaces that the forcibly-removed left behind. Apartheid was lived every day, every night; passes restricted the movement of non-whites/non-citizens into white-only areas, which were segregated in their racially 'pure' and gated affluence. And threaded through all of this was the apartheid psyche, which lingers on in some quarters, as we will show. As Lefebvre observes, to change space is to change life.

Let it not be imaged that only South Africa was involved in these oppressive and exploitative spatial racial practices. For they developed in collusion with British oriented colonial and racial capitalism which began in the later 1790s when the Dutch East India Company failed, when the 'The Cape' becomes a British colony and when the London Missionary Society set up its first station. These exploitative spatial racial practices intensified when, in the 1880s, gold and other minerals were discovered, the powerful mining and energy sectors began and the use of 'unfree back labor' became systemic (Terreblanche 2012b).

And in 2012, nearly two decades after the official end of apartheid (1994) and of the hoped-for brighter days of 'democratization', 'transformation' and 'rainbow politics', the sad legacy of all this remains intertwined with some significant differences. The new black ANC government, the minerals/energy complex, and American pressure groups developed what has become known as 'the elite compromise' and South Africa became part of the, perhaps now fading a little, American-led neo-liberal global empire. A small, new black elite and middle class emerged, local and foreign corporations profited handsomely but the economic-spatial segregation of the impoverished black majority remained.

Poverty, unemployment and inequality continued as a lived socio-spatial practice of deprivation made worse by the AIDS/HIV pandemic and by massive inward migration to the cities from the rural 'homelands' and from other African countries and the resulting emergence of 'informal settlements' or 'squatter camps' which lack even the most basic infrastructure. Overall, income inequality has *increased* since 1994 and South Africa is amongst the most unequal societies in the world (Terreblanche 2012a).

But none of this is visible from Greystone whose gracious buildings and fragrant grounds contrast starkly with the cramped and dusty (in summer) or dank (in winter) spaces of the townships and settlements; 'the tastes, textures, smells, sights and sounds' of which are so poignantly described by Dlamini (2010). Greystone is located in expensive, pleasant, quiet, hillside suburbs well above and well away from the cramped and noisy quarters of the poor. For most of its 140 years spatial and social distancing have happily coincided and ensured a sensual field unspoilt and undisturbed by the bodies, sounds and smells of the abject elsewhere. Over time, old and new campus architecture, design, aesthetics and acoustics have been manicured to reflect and provoke tasteful and tangible elite sensibilities. Stately old buildings, elegant gardens, deliberately hushed courtyards with soothing fountains, pristine playing fields and tennis courts, impeccable state-of-the-art 'creative centers' and science buildings, for instance, are solid markers and makers of distinction and entitlement. They feed alumni nostalgia, parental ambitions and student aspirations. They express privilege and signal possibility (Fig. 4).

Always an elite private school for privileged white girls (with the occasional exception) it has now 'democratized' and opened its gates to privileged 'black', 'Asian' and 'Colored' girls from South Africa, other countries in Africa and a small

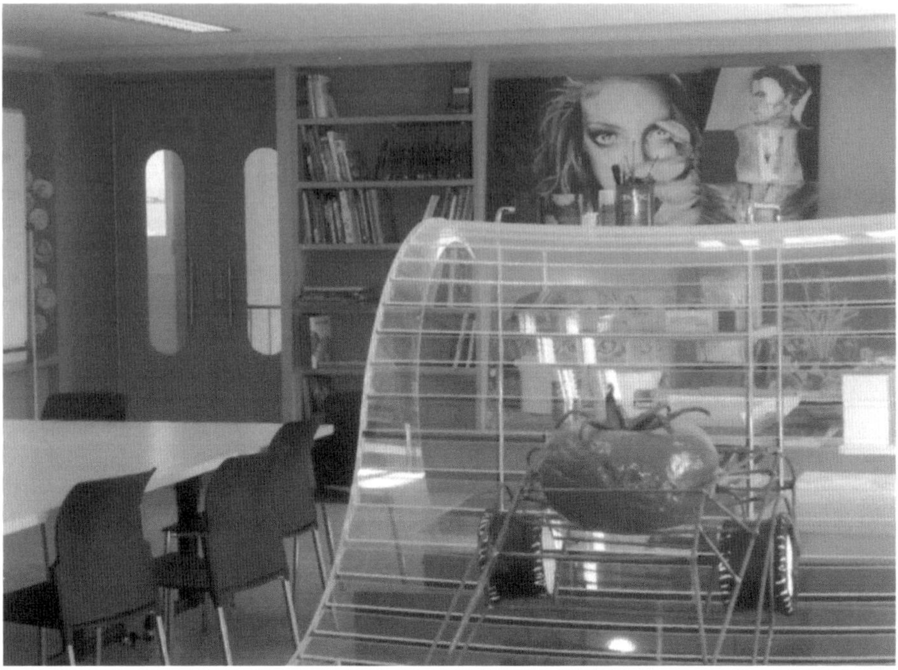

Fig. 4 A pristine Greystone classroom

numbers of black girls on scholarships. These girls are now inside the exquisite spaces of distinction from which they once would have been excluded. But are they now outsiders within (Fig. 5)?

The boarding house population is now predominantly black. In a discussion with Jane and Debbie a set of Old Girls in their 70s and 80s identified some problems with this. Shirley said ‘Some very nice children who want to be boarders won’t come here because they don’t want to be in a black boarding house. Not because there is anything wrong with these black children, but just because they can’t make friends with [them]’. The social difficulties, she and others remarked on, stem from having ‘nothing in common’ and ‘they’re very noisy’. The notion of ‘very noisy’ developed quickly into a critical discussion of life in black townships such as Khayelitsha, and of white students and their parents being uncomfortable socializing with students from there. Going to such spaces in the city was clearly out of the question.

For white families who don’t want their daughters in Greystone’s (black) boarding house, geographical location becomes a proxy for discrimination. As the following remark from Jan indicates it is used to justify the choice of a different elite private school for girls:

> It’s the distance, the geography…it’s just because of the hellish roads today. It makes a very long day for a …day girl, and this is the area of the southern suburbs where people can afford independent schools, you have Herschel, you have Springfield, you have got Rustenburg.

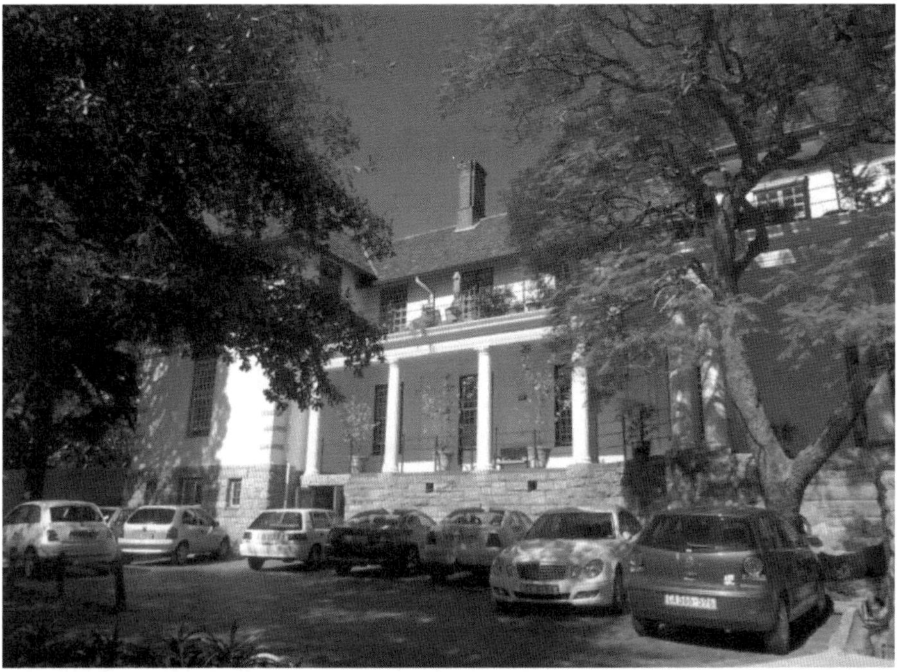

Fig. 5 The post-colonial colonnades and cars of Greystone

Clearly there are ways in which elite private schools can still be used to avoid democratization along racial lines.

Securitization

Private security companies have increased enormously in both nations since the 1990s. This growth has coincided with democratic reforms as well as the cycles of neo-liberal reforms that have slowly seen personal security as something to be augmented, rather than in the hands of the state.

This development is, of course, global in its scale. But unlike most nations in the North, Argentina and South Africa both have had recent examples of civil unrest that have justified moneyed interests increasing their defenses in line with their perceived fears. Moreover both nations have a history of social unrest that preceded the rise of ubiquitous security industry. Nevertheless, at both schools as well as the homes of the students, there are social aesthetics that include measures of security that extend from the subtle—surreptitious guards and CCTV—to the carapace—barbed-wire fences and bullet-proof glass.

The paradox, however, is that during the same time the school fences have become more porous. As the schools' eliteness has grown in the last couple of decades, the entry of other social groups—black and poor students on scholarships—has increased. This change stems directly from the liberal revolutions that South Africa and Argentina have undergone. Lefebrve's perceived (spatial practices) spaces of design interacted directly with the way that the space is lived (spaces of representation). And so here the social aesthetics of the school includes means of surveillance and exclusion alongside a welcoming attitude toward those from previously suspect social groups. Such welcoming is controlled, of course; anyone can't just stroll in. Nevertheless, the illusion of liberalism's equality, in these cases as elsewhere, becomes apparent.

Security from/for Whom?

In a highly planned manner, the South African police state of apartheid certainly protected white property and privilege. Even so during the apartheid regime property and privilege were also privately securitized behind heavily locked gates and high walls often topped with spikes, glass or barbed wire.

The freedom of movement for the non-white populations that emerged after the 1994 democratic elections, the additional demands on the state for a range of things beyond securing white power, the failure of the ANC to address issues of poverty all left the white wealthy minority feeling just as, if not more, vulnerable than before. Having had to 'voluntarily' give up their monopoly on political power they were additionally eager to protect their private property. This, the rise of the black elite and middle class, also demanding security, and the user pays regime of neoliberalism led to an explosion in the private security industry, more armed security guards, more alarm systems, more sophisticated security arrangements. In Cape Town security dominates the use of space and the ways that life is lived—at least for the wealthy (Fig. 6).

In the post-apartheid state the privileged feel less secure, not just because of the high crime rates (which are much higher in the poorer parts of the city) but because they are the minority beneficiaries of a state that facilitates such vast gaps between rich and poor. Acknowledged as indefensible by critics of South Africa's elite settlement and of its high Gini coefficient, their privilege seems more in need of defending. This is not surprising given that in 2008 the richest 10 million received almost 75 % of the total income while the poorest 25 million received less than 8 % (Terreblanche 2012a).

Like all the nearby schools, Greystone's gates are fortified at all times by two guards. They must approve day-to-day entry. At this school barriers have come down as some previously abjectified students from near and far trickle in and climb up, but other barriers have gone up simultaneously. Black guards are used to defend white privilege and barbed wire is prettily concealed in the bougainvillea at a fence line (Fig. 7).

On other sides of the city, and indeed the country, in the townships and informal settlements where space is often out of control, 'security' is much less of an issue

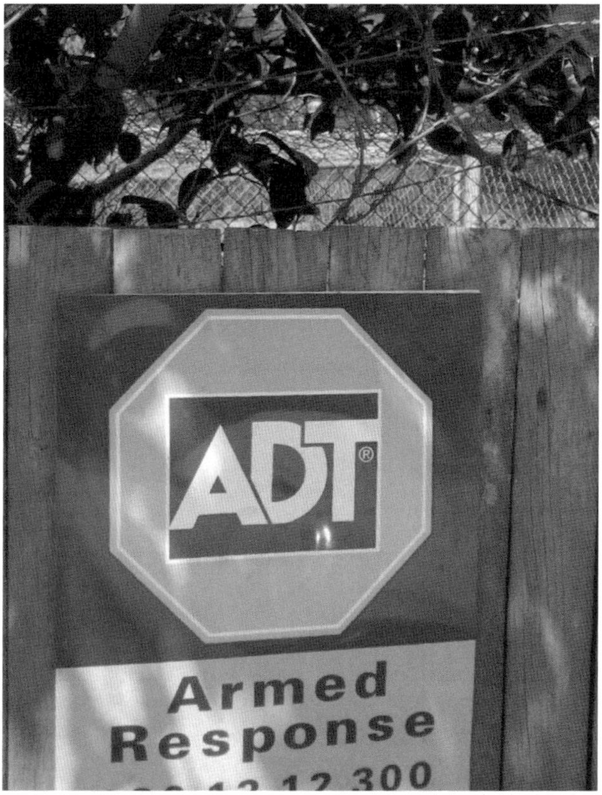

Fig. 6 Armed guards are only a call away in Cape Town

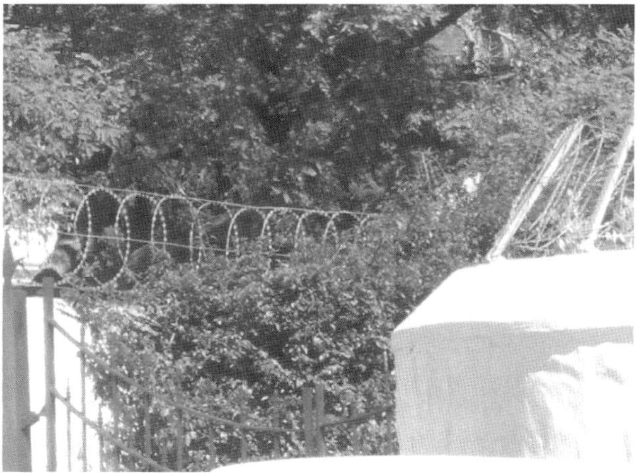

Fig. 7 Razor wire adorns substantial walls of a South African residence

than the provision of basic services; public housing, power and water. Like South Africa's shockingly poorly paid but organized workers, who have engaged in wave after wave of strike action over recent years, the unemployed poor and informal workers too have regularly protested with a vengeance. Township and community protests have become common (Dwyer and Zeilig 2012). The Abahlali baseMjondolo (the shack-dwellers' movement) campaigns relentlessly against evictions and for public housing. And when services are not officially provided, they provide them for themselves stringing up unofficial power lines. For them all, as for Lefebvre, space is a very political matter. They refuse to be determined by space and, in the case of informal settlers, they occupy spaces even when none is available for them (Fig. 8).

In August of 2012, while Jane and Debbie were in Cape Town, protesters were demanding such 'service delivery' basics. They blocked the N2 to the airport and flights from Cape Town International Airport were delayed. They marched in the city bowl taking their protests to the provincial and city governments, claiming their right to be central in central urban space. In the settlements and townships they throw petrol bombs and stones and burnt tyres. Drawing on slogans of the anti-apartheid era, they threatened to make the province 'ungovernable'. The press said 'Protests cripple Cape Town' (Bester 2012). But in Greystone and its neighboring suburbs there was peace, quiet and privilege-as-usual.

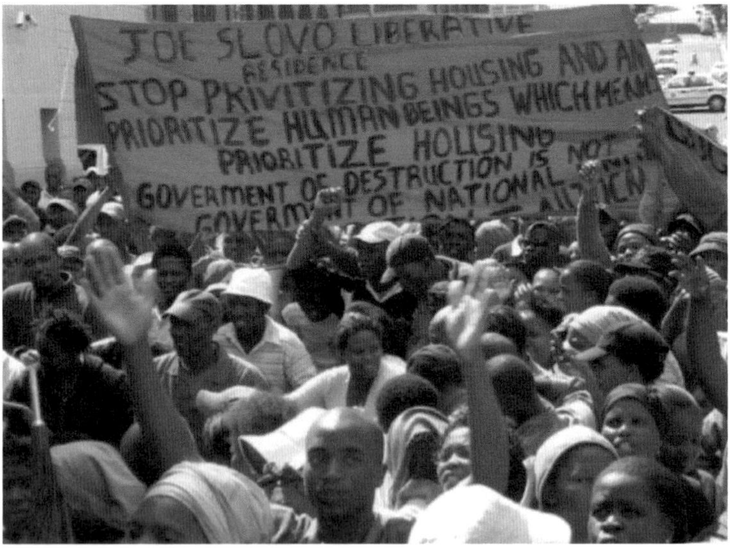

Fig. 8 Housing protest. (This photo has been altered into black and white from the original by FromBelow, 'Joe Slovo at Capetown High Court,' December 2007 via Wikipedia, Creative Commons Attribution)

Private Eyes

In the case of Latin America, it has been argued that the fear behind such security concern is a direct outcome of the fears created by the uncertainty of the dictatorship years. Soon after the end of these times, sociologist Emilio Mignone outlined how the wake of such repression has stymied the faith in the public sphere (Mignone 1992). This lack of faith, simultaneous with the neo-liberal revolution, inflated belief in private provision. The fear surrounding the possibility of kidnapping, roving death squads, or random violence perpetrated by both state and militant groups of all stripes was, with the return of democracy, quickly diverted into new concerns about threats to personal wealth during years of new economic opportunity. This fits neatly into Buenos Aires citizens' perpetuation of discourses of insecurity in the last couple of decades (Kessler 2009).

In terms of the Caledonian School, the security is ever-present, but not overwhelmingly threatening. The front gates of the school are relatively understated. This situation keeps with a common desire for a low profile (*bajo perfil*) expressed by the school community.[4] As the image here portrays, the school is policed at all times by besuited guards who are obvious during school hours, less so at other times. A system of gates and doors with buzzers and cameras allowed entry to the school at limited points (Fig. 9).

[4] The description speaks of a downplaying of wealth or disproving of extravagant displays of wealth. It also can be read as meaning not bringing attention to the economic elite that the school serves. Engagement with the public sphere—in formal politics, for example—is regarded as corrupting or distasteful. The likely historical reason for this lies in the unpredictable nature of doing business in a nation with a long history of social unrest.

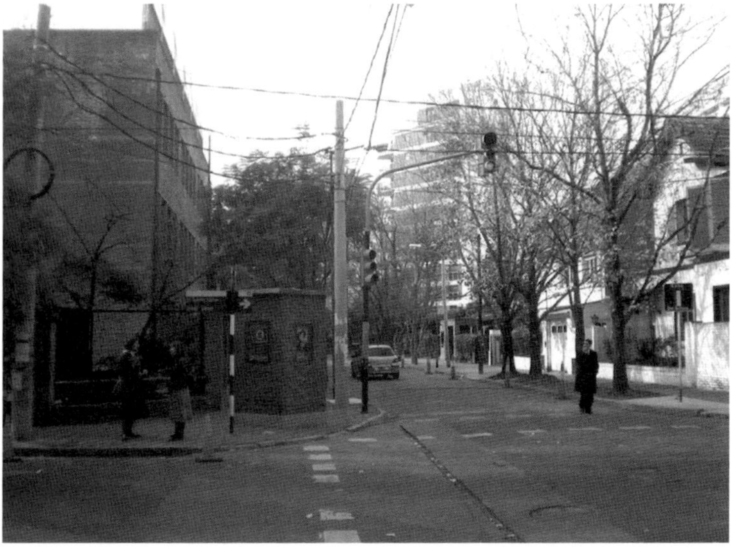

Fig. 9 Caledonian Front Gates

Again, this is not uncommon in private schools in Latin America or elsewhere around the world for that matter. The neighborhood in which the Caledonian School currently sits is filled with private sentinels on every second or third corner of the suburb—they are paid by the inhabitants of the area mostly, it seemed, to watch television and kick the bitumen around their small huts.

What Howard found especially interesting about the security guards at the school is that they knew what was happening each day. The school was an extremely busy place and so the guards had a running list of the day's events—some were routine, such as school arrivals and departures; others were less so, such as visiting schools, excursions, and other events provided outside of school hours. And yet, these figures that guarded the school were not privy to the world that they protected. They held the line between the worlds of the privileged and the world of the everyday Argentine. For this reason they were highly valued. But they were not afforded the opportunity to send their children to the school. Instead they were included in the friendly atmosphere of the workplace in which such class lines remain unsaid.

Still, as anyone who has observed private security guards, or perhaps may have been one, knows, theirs' is a space of responsibility for power that also includes a degree of autonomy—for the lived experiences of camaraderie and, if nothing else, boredom—as they are simultaneously separated from that which they protect. In this sense, the gates of these schools, and those who monitor them, capture the three aspects of Lefebrve's spatial interpretation: how they are conceived, perceived, and lived.

Outsiders Within

Urban theorists have long argued that social divisions will likely increase in cities during the twenty-first century. Such an increase is counterintuitive to the spread of liberal governance throughout the world in the last few decades. Security measures, the markers of division, are just one symptom of this trend among the wealthy. For the majority on the other side of the fences the manifestations need more than protective measures—with insecurity around food, health, and education set to intensify. The global tendency is thus toward urban societies fracturing along racial/class lines with the likelihood of worsening urban conflicts (Davis 2006).

All of this has taken place under the auspices of liberal market expansion, under the sign of globalization, without affording the political rights previously affiliated with its logic. Segregated urban spaces struggle to house even semblances of civil society. At the upper echelons of this social model ties deepen between political leadership and social elites who are increasingly removed from the larger population both economically and geographically. These beneficiaries of neo-liberal globalization are almost immune to its social devastation.

In the nation states discussed here, such processes are grafted to their histories. South Africa's post-apartheid situation has seen the de facto continuation of previously codified racial divides through economic means. Economic reforms tend to favor already landed white South Africans, but so too those within the rising black middle class. Similarly, in Argentina the process of Latin-Americanization, a coming to terms with the presence of poverty and class divides, which has been going on for at least four decades, has begun to see race—especially Latin American indigeneity—emerge as an issue within existing discussions of class (Ko 2013).[5]

Yet the divisions are not impermeable. Contradictions remain that expose how space is used to engage fellow citizens. Lefebrve's spatial triad elucidates this dynamic by recognizing that the built environment becomes a site of power relations through its different uses. Elite schools exemplify this process. Social hierarchy is present in the way individuals use the space. The presence of 'support staff,' for example, is an important contributor to the social aesthetics of any elite space. Some people learn in the school; others clean it. Both acts are of a different order of social performance and thus define actors as well as the space in relation to larger social contexts.

The tolerance of outsiders within—workers or guests—accentuates the informal segregation of urban spaces more generally: the exception that proves the rule. As we have shown, high fees and high fences provide exclusivity; but the situation, as always, is more complicated than that. There is a temptation to see the schools like the closed neighborhoods in which many of their students live. To do so would be a disservice to the recent historical and political changes. The rhetoric of inclusivity exhorts the schools to be more permeable than the closed neighborhoods because they represent liberal institutions *par excellence*. This fact alone demands some degree of social engagement to claim to be so.[6]

In the case of both our schools, promoting an inclusive ethos is a genuine goal, especially insofar as the administration and teaching staff want not to be seen as elitist. They are, more importantly, highly attuned to the liberalizing discourses of global education as well as local politics. The internal message of the school to its charges—via the curriculum and the school values (read ideology)—is one of inclusion. The paradox is patent, however. The clientele of the schools is usually contributing to the social inequity via entrepreneurship or professions that facilitate ongoing social divisions (as well as allow them to pay the school fees). This paradox is the main social problem for such schools. Moreover, we would suggest, it is symptomatic of liberal democracies at the current conjuncture, especially those fledglings, which have hitched their political futures to the market logic at odds with inclusivity. In other words, just like the societies of which they are apart, elite schools like Greystone and Caledonian are representative of broader spatially designated forms of social division. The result, in social aesthetics terms, is schools that accommodate the use of their space with a lip service to such exclusionary inclusivity.

[5] That race is an issue in Argentina at all still seems a surprise to some. It is a testament the success of nationalist homogenization and the control of the past. Scholars now working to rectify the record will no doubt meet with resistance.

[6] Coming to terms with the inclusive nature of social discourse has been a common trait among elite schools in our larger project 'Elite Independent Schools in Globalizing Circumstances.' The openness that a liberal education affords does not always sit easily with the exclusionary expense it incurs (see Khan 2011).

Open-Handed Gestures

Since 2001, Argentina finds itself in the odd situation, especially to an outside observer, of becoming Latin American. This shift has an historical explanation that requires some elaboration. Suffice it to say that Argentina's Latin-Americanization can be read, on the one hand, as the nation's coming to terms with its location in the continent, rather than pining for a European past. On the other hand, it is also used as a lament for the visible presence of poverty in the streets of Buenos Aires, in a way that replicated other South American capitals. Part of this was linked to the insecurity in the city—an insecurity that is both real and imagined.

For the Caledonian School this shift has also coincided with its move from a school associated with the British community to one that is now almost exclusively catering to the very wealthy members of society. As such there is a need to see the school as being Argentine through and through, albeit with a slightly disdainful attitude to the educational requirements of the state, as well as not reinforcing a popular image of its elitist nature. One way of achieving this is through connections to those outside the gates of the school. Connections have been made with other schools in the area as well as in other parts of the Province of Buenos Aires (Fig. 10).

There is also recognition of those outsiders that are integral to the school's functioning: those who contribute to the social aesthetics not just through their labors but their very presence. The school held an open day for the families of support staff—cleaners, cooks, and security guards, all of which are hired through private

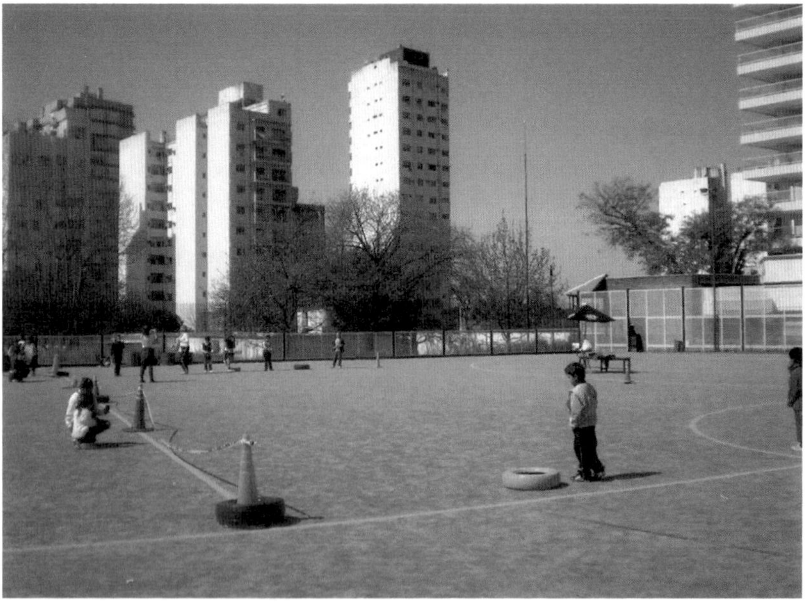

Fig. 10 The Astroturf field at Caledonian during a family day

firms and thus not strictly members of the school's community. Speaking to some of the families on the day, they expressed their enthusiasm for the event put on. Most families I chatted with were Argentine, with some from migrant backgrounds in Paraguay. The children were especially happy with the fun on offer—face painting, games, and bouncing castles. These kids' experiences of school would be vastly different from those at Caledonian, not least contrasting spaces. These grounds of the Caledonian School are not vast (its playing fields are located elsewhere) but they are certainly luxurious compared to the typical *patio* of a public school in Buenos Aires. Usually the *patio* a confined concrete space for playing that the children maximize in its use (Fig. 11).

The open day could be read in two equally revealing ways. First, there was a sense that the day opened the facilities of the school, and the joy of the teaching staff, to those who support them in their daily work. This is an honorable sentiment and not one that should be dismissed with cynicism. It was a family fun day that was relatively new and quite different from anything that the school had offered in the past. As a spatial practice, the school was being used as a site of social intimacy between as range of social groups—the working classes of the support staff, the middle classes of the teaching staff, and the upper-class families who sent their kids

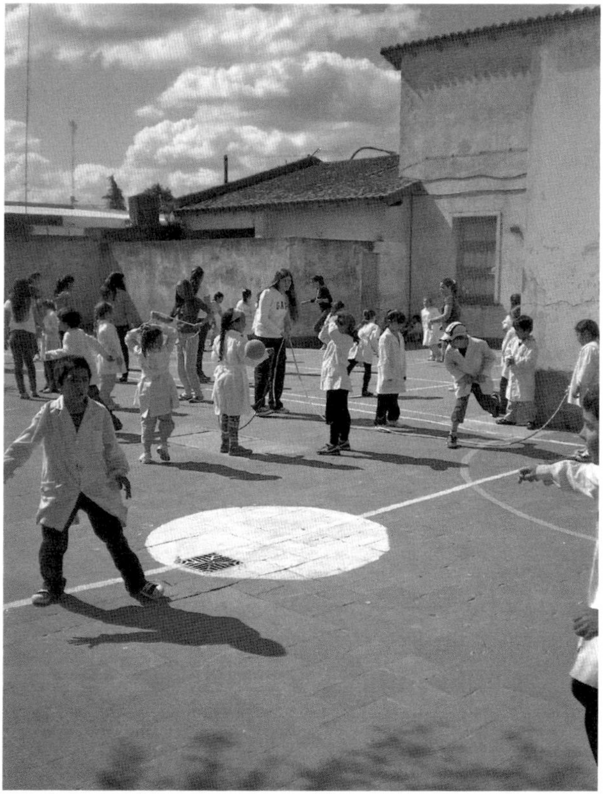

Fig. 11 A typical play area in an Argentine public school

to Caledonian (which was, it has to be said, the most under-represented group). 'There should be more events like this,' said one teacher to Howard on the day. 'This represents the future of the school, the direction that it is going in. Hopefully more events like this will happen. It is disappointing that there aren't more students here today.'[7]

Which leads us to such gesture's limits. The running of a school requires so many logistical arrangements, in which the support staff is crucial, that to have a single day, or afternoon, of gratitude can be seen as really an elaborate display of class condescension or, more kindly, class guilt. Creating ties between members of a school community requires much more—at the heart of which is access to the education provided.

The Limits of Elite Liberalism

Greystone's most significant and long lasting tradition is the annual Founders Day procession in which all the girls and professional staff walk from the school through the central city bowl to the St George's Anglican Cathedral for a service and then return to the school for an afternoon tea. The procession's leaders hold high the school's traditional ceremonial banners. The numbers swell as many ex-students and parents join the procession. When it eventually arrives at the Cathedral, waiting-in-welcome are significant figures from the church as well as rows of elderly 'Old Girls'. This is a formal ritual. Hair braids and full school uniform are required for all girls, hats and frocks are preferred for adult women and key figures of the church are in full ceremonial dress.

This event speaks to the school's long links with the Anglican Church and, by inference, its British connections. These links date back to the school's foundation by the first Anglican Bishop of Cape Town in 1871. Since then the school has constantly asserted that it is 'firmly centered in the Anglican faith', although in an undated newsletter (probably in 2010 or 2011) it said 'Whilst the Anglican Faith is a cornerstone of our ethos, we actively welcome, encourage and embrace every religion and faith amongst our learners. The world is a diverse ecosystem and our passion is celebrating diversity and 'teaching for life''.

The Cathedral is most famous for being the home of Nobel Laureate Archbishop Desmond Tutu (in place from 1986–1996) who was particularly close to the school's

[7] *There was an added layer to this* day. Another part of the school was open to other young people, mostly girls, who were competing in a Scottish festival of dance and song. (Scottish dancing is fashionable among the private schools for reasons no one could explain beyond tartan skirts.) Although not an official school event, the occasion did have a more than tangential relationship to the Scottish origins of the Caledonian school. Much like a tango *milonga* in Edinburgh, the festivities showed global culture in full garb. But more tellingly, when viewed in concert with the family fun day at the other end of the campus, it showed two different manifestations of the school culture: its past and its future in the present. Spatially, the whole arrangement—which could simply be seen as a matter of allocation—captures Lefebrve's point about the complicated way that space is lived and the richness of the social aesthetics that results.

previous principal (in place from 1990–2007). Together they were responsible for many of the school's more liberal and progressive ideas and practices, one aim being to help to produce leaders for the *new democratic* South Africa. One of these is the 'Girl child in Afrika' campaign which awards bursaries for 'girl-children in Africa who would otherwise not be able to afford an education such as offered by 'Greystone' School'.

> The basic principle underpinning this project is the belief that these learners will be grown and developed in such a way that they will go out into the world and make a meaningful difference to the future of our society (Undated school newsletter).

Of this project, Archbishop Emeritus Tutu said

> 'Greystone' is a school which has consciously striven for excellence without elitism and has achieved this delicate balance. Greystone is educating young women to celebrate themselves and their responsibility in a radically changing South Africa. I congratulate the school on their efforts to be as inclusive as possible in offering places to the daughters of families who cannot afford the standard of education the school offers. (Undated school Newsletter)

This Founders' Day ritual is likely to, consciously or unconsciously, confirm the girls' sense that they are, indeed, members of Cape Town's establishment. The beautiful Company Gardens, they stroll through, are bordered by Government Avenue on one side and Queen Victoria street on the other. They pass close-by many significant municipal and cultural buildings including the Provincial Parliament building, the High Court Library, the South African museum, a campus of the University of Cape Town and monuments to Cecil Rhodes. History is inscribed in this space of dominance and this history can be excavated.

Collectively these streets, buildings and monuments express South Africa's colonial, apartheid and post-apartheid history, they are material signifiers of power and powerful upheavals. For example Rhodes is best known for his ambition to extend British imperialism from 'Cape to Cairo', for opening up the hugely profitable diamond mines and for his ruthless and cruel treatments of forced black labour. On the other hand the Cathedral is a reminder of Archbishop Tutu's moral courage and social activism. This is, then, a space of multiple signifiers; of South Africa's terrible oppressions, of its democratic liberation and of its current failings. For it is also a space where service delivery protest rallies are held (Fig. 12).

In 2010, when Jane and Debbie joined the procession, we noticed that, as most school members left the school grounds, black members of its domestic and ground staff, some dressed in special purple outfits for the day, remained behind. They stood on the stairs and waved farewell; smiling. For some time they had been cooking, cleaning and primping the buildings and grounds in preparation for this event. Vases of exquisite flowers graced each corner. The trestles with their white tablecloths they laid ready as the rest of the school departed and on their return these were heavy with food and drink. Parents assembled and moved into friendship groups but white and black parents largely stayed apart. The following day, the head of the kitchen attended the school assembly and received a standing ovation. She was wearing her special purple uniform again (Fig. 13).

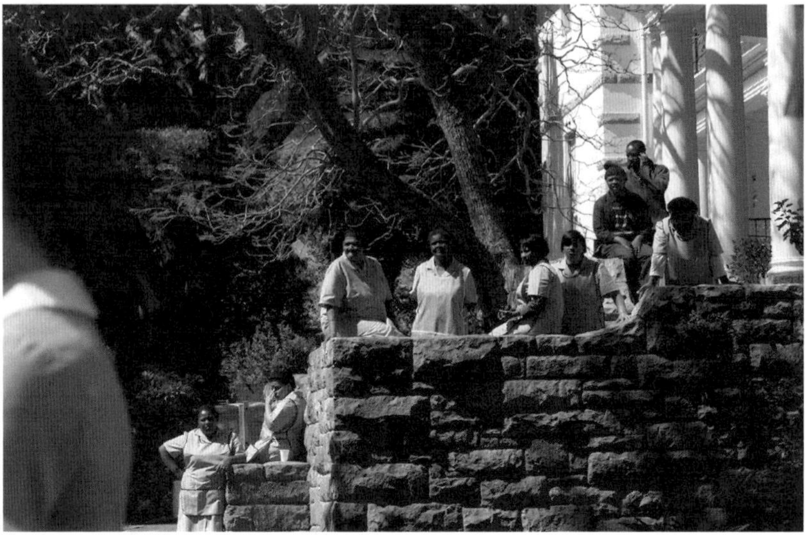

Fig. 12 Greystone's domestic and grounds staff not attending the Founders' Day procession

These are the most poignant moments of this event for they indicated the limits of the school's liberalism and of democratic South Africa. The applause felt like gratuitous gratitude and we wondered will it ever be possible for the whole school staff to walk through the city together, black manual workers with the city's current and future elite. Tutu congratulated the school for being as *'inclusive as possible'*. But it seems unable to make a gesture that transcends race and class together. We have been left wondering, if it were to happen, what such a gesture would it signify and what else might follow?

Fig. 13 Trestle tables prepared for the Greystone's Founders' Day celebrations

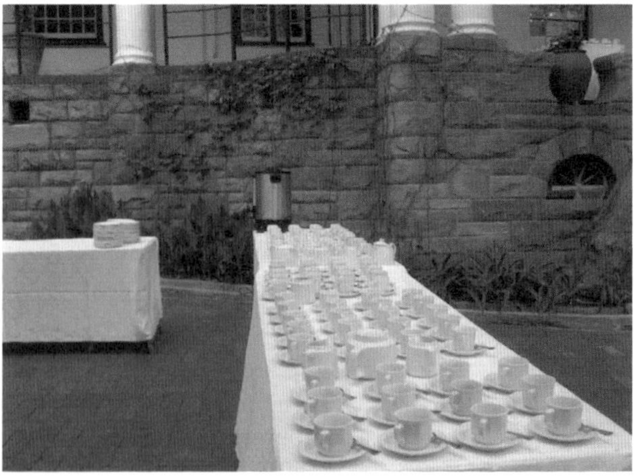

This ritual in the conceived and lived spaces of the school and the city offers highly ambiguous signals. It indicates that the girls are destined for leadership of some sort, that they are expected to 'make a meaningful difference to the future of our society'. But 'what difference?' Will they be part of the ongoing 'elite compromise' mentioned earlier or will they respond to Tutu's assertion that:

> If you are neutral in situations of injustice, you have chosen the side of the oppressor. If an elephant has its foot on the tail of a mouse and you say that you are neutral, the mouse will not appreciate your neutrality. (Quigley 2003, p. 8)

After all, under their noses, the school's manual workers, labor largely unnoticed, and travel each long day to and from the city's under resourced townships where unemployment, poverty and crime are rampant. If Lefebrve is right and perceived space is where radical potential resides might the girls be encouraged to perceive this space of the city in another way? Might they be provoked to ask why they have the 'right to the city' (Lefebvre 1996) and why so many others do not? Might they then consider how to produce space differently and more justly?

Conclusion

Our examples of these two schools' social aesthetics, working with Lefebrve's framework, reveal the ways that historical changes redefine privileged spaces without necessarily challenging entrenched interests. Or, to put it another way, how social elites are able to control spaces, like elite private schools, to benefit their own class interests. There are certainly differences between the current ways that the schools produce space and those in pre-democratic periods. And there are also challenges to these class interests in both nations. But the point is that the groups that these schools cater to—economic and professional elites, by and large—continue to assert their position of superior wealth, and by association cultural superiority, through security measures or through carefully orchestrated interactions with other social classes and races.

The production of space creates specific social aesthetics that facilitate inclusion and exclusion. This has to do with the ownership of the space, its design, and its history; but in everyday life there is a specific affect that occurs. This affect, of the pattern created by their repetition in particular spaces, contributes to the social aesthetics. In a school we see classes taking place, but there is also much else that is unacknowledged. In an elite school there are certain signifiers in the make up of the space—rooms decorated with tradition, for example—or rituals that occur to give life to the space. It is here that Lefebrve's spatial triad illuminates the concept of social aesthetics.

In our two settings, the social aesthetics of the schools differ and overlap according to specific and shared histories. The issue of race is more pronounced in one than the other; class is a concern in both. Although Atlantically-divided, the schools share a British public school heritage in an antipodean setting. But today, in contemporary globalizing circumstances, the schools are arguably more aligned. This is certainly the case when it comes to developments around the need for elite schools to be more inclusive while simultaneously excluding others through rising fees and securitization. As a result, these British-tradition elite schools cultivate spaces with closely aligned social aesthetics. Their students would likely feel more at home on each other's campuses than in other parts of their cities.

References

Bester, J. (2012). Protests cripple Cape Town. IOL News. http://www.iol.co.za/news/south-africa/western-cape/protests-cripple-cape-town-1.1360307. Accessed 11 Aug 2012.

Bond, P. (2005). *Elite transition: From apartheid to neoliberalism in South Africa*. Scottsville: University of KwaZulu-Natal Press.

Davis, M. (2006). *Planet of slums*. London: Verso.

Dlamini, J. (2010). *Native nostalgia*. Aukland Park: Jacana Media.

Dwyer, P., & Zeilig, L. (2012). *African struggles today: Social movements since independence*. Chicago: Haymarket Books.

Kessler, G. (2009). *El sentimiento de inseguridad: sociología del temor al delito*. Buenos Aires: Siglo Veintiuno Editores.

Khan, S. R. (2011). *Privilege: The making of an adolescent elite at St. Paul' school*. Princeton: Princeton University Press.

Ko, C. T. (2013). From whiteness to diversity: Crossing the racial threshold in bicentennial Argentina. Ethnic and Racial Studies. www.tandfonline.com/doi/abs/10.1080/01419870.2013.835056. Accessed 31 Dec 2013.

Lefebvre, H. (1991). Production of space. Oxford: Wiley Blackwell.

Lefebvre, H. (1996). The right to the city. In E. Kofman & E. Lebas (Eds.), *Writings on cities* (pp. 147–159). Oxford: Blackwell.

MacDougall, D. (1999). Social aesthetics and the Doon school. *Visual Anthropology Review, 15*(1), 3–20.

Mignone, E. F. (1992). Beyond fear: Forms of justice and compensation. In J. E. Corradi, P. W. Fagen, & M. A. Garretón (Eds.), *Fear at the edge: State terror and resistance in Latin America* (pp. 250–266). Berkeley: University of California Press.

Narodowski, M., & Andrada, M. (2001). The privatization of education in Argentina. *Journal of Education Policy, 16*(6), 585–595.

Quigley, W. P. (2003). *Ending poverty as we know it: Guaranteeing a right to a job at a living wage*. Philadelphia: Temple University Press.

Shields, R. (1999). *Lefebrve, love and struggle: Spatial dialectics*. London: Routledge.

Terreblanche, S. (2012a). *Lost in transformation: South Africa's search for a new future since 1986*. Sandtown: KMM Review Publishing Company.

Terreblanche, S. (2012b). *A history of inequality in South Africa, 1652–2002*. Scottsville: University of KwaZulu-Natal Press.

Jane Kenway is Australian Research Council Professorial Fellow, Professor of Global Education Studies at Monash University, Australia, and an elected Fellow of the Academy of Social Sciences, Australia. Her research expertise is in socio-cultural studies of education in the context of wider social and cultural change. Her more recent jointly edited books are *Asia as Method in Education Studies: A Defiant Research Imagination*, (Routledge 2015) and *Globalising the Research Imagination* (Routledge 2009). Her more recent jointly written books are *Masculinity*

Beyond the Metropolis (Palgrave 2006) and *Haunting the Knowledge Economy* (Routledge 2006). She has published numerous book chapters and journal articles. She leads the international team conducting the research project called *Elite independent schools in globalising circumstances: a multi-sited global ethnography.*

Howard Prosser researches and teaches at the Faculty of Education, Monash University, Australia. He has taught history in Australian secondary schools and universities. His research interests include Social Theory, History of Ideas, and Ethnography. Most recently he has been working on a study of political culture at an elite school in Argentina.

Visual Essay: Space

Johannah Fahey

Inside & Outside

Old Cloisters in the commercial center of Bridgetown is overshadowed by the Tom Adams Financial Centre building, which houses the Central Bank of Barbados, the national monetary authority advising the Government of Barbados. In Hong Kong, a city that is an international financial centre, the construction of apartment buildings around Cathedral College continues unabated, real estate in this neighborhood is at a premium nowadays as a new subway stop has just been completed. At Founders in Australia, the school's colonnade frames the high-rise apartment buildings beyond the school grounds, some of which are home to the international students that have selected this school out of a globalizing elite school market. In Cyprus, the green line that separates North from South, Greek Cypriot from Turkish Cypriot, is guarded by the military, at the Lefkos Academy there are also barriers at the entrance but this is a place where both Greek and Turkish Cypriot students come together. In Buenos Aires, the construction of the Caledonian School's new campus, situated near the *barrio privados*, or private neighborhoods, in the north, is well underway. The school's northward shift is in keeping with the ongoing trend among the wealthy to move further north of the city where security is supposedly greater. Continuing class divisions are explicitly alluded to by the word '*Justicia*' scrawled on a city wall. In India, the world just beyond Ripon College's walls is one where space is a luxury that most cannot afford, and where the polluted air is filled with the constant sound of car horns and traffic. In contrast empty space and relative quiet abound inside the school grounds. At Greystone the 'armed response' from security is a warning to perceived threats that exist beyond the school's fortified walls. While in a South African township, makeshift fences are built from savaged scrap metal.

J. Fahey (✉)
Monash University, Melbourne, Australia
e-mail: johannah.fahey@monash.edu

J. Fahey et al. (eds.), *In the Realm of the Senses,* Cultural Studies and Transdisciplinarity in Education, DOI 10.1007/978-981-287-350-7_4

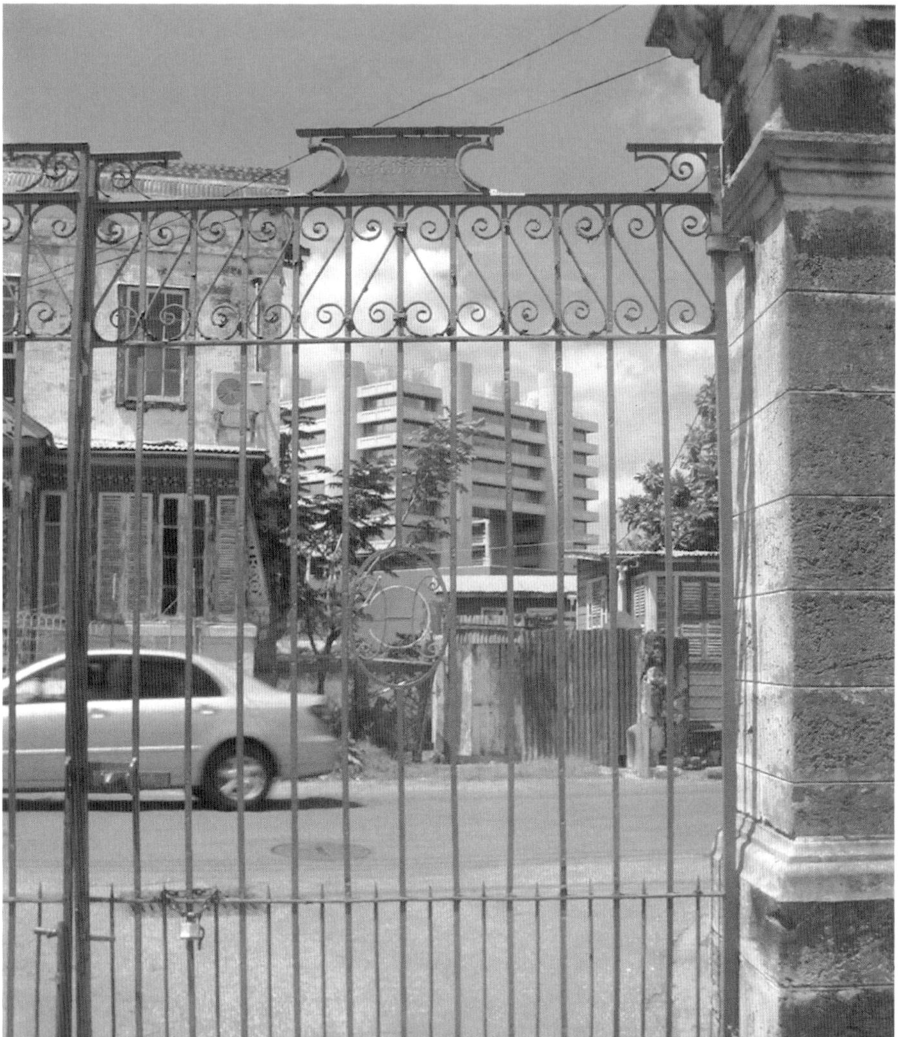

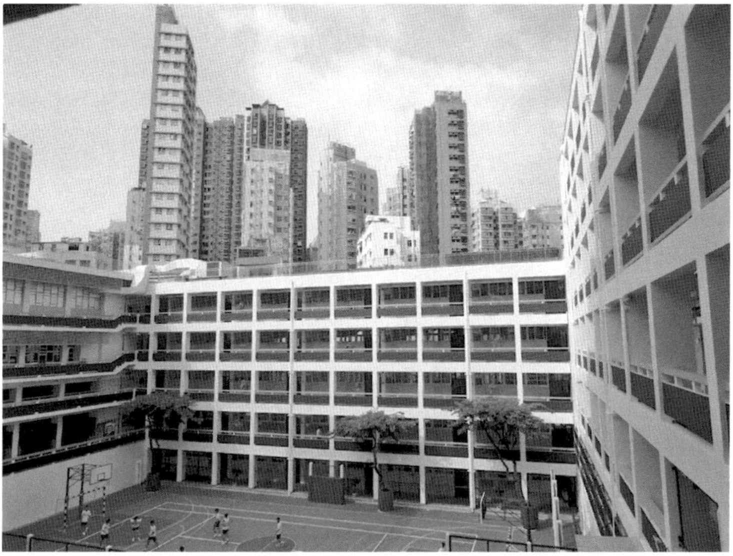

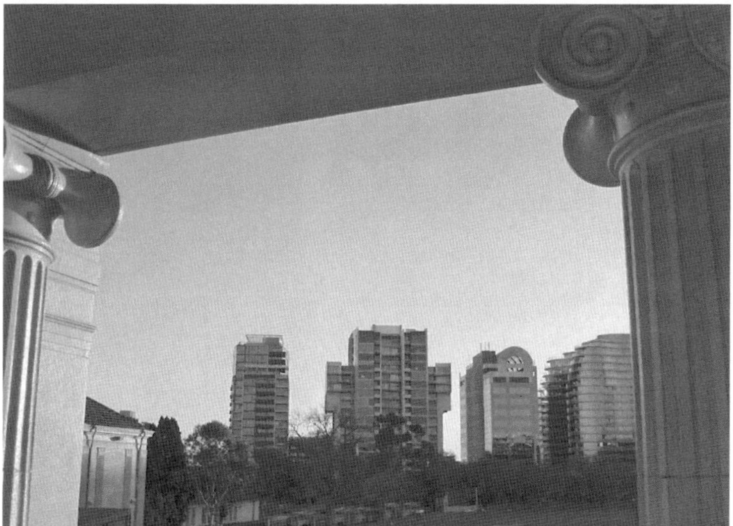

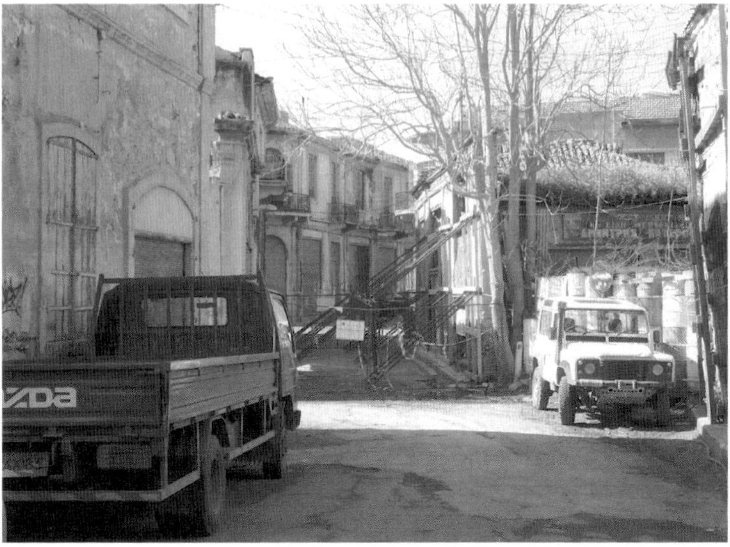
ZDA

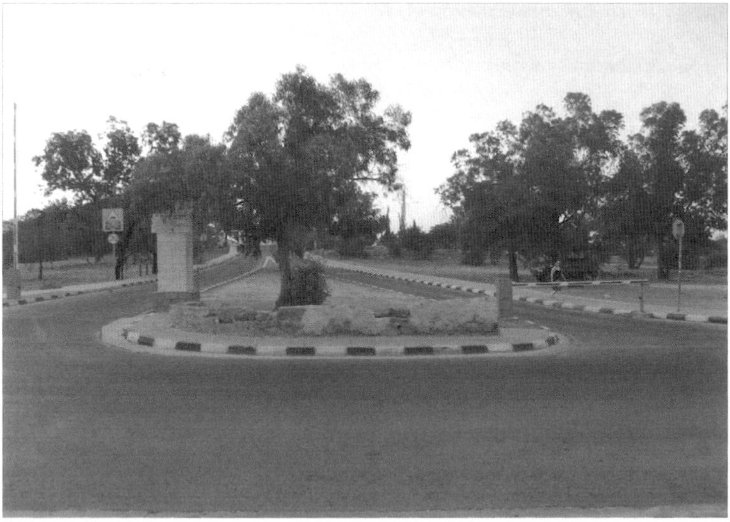

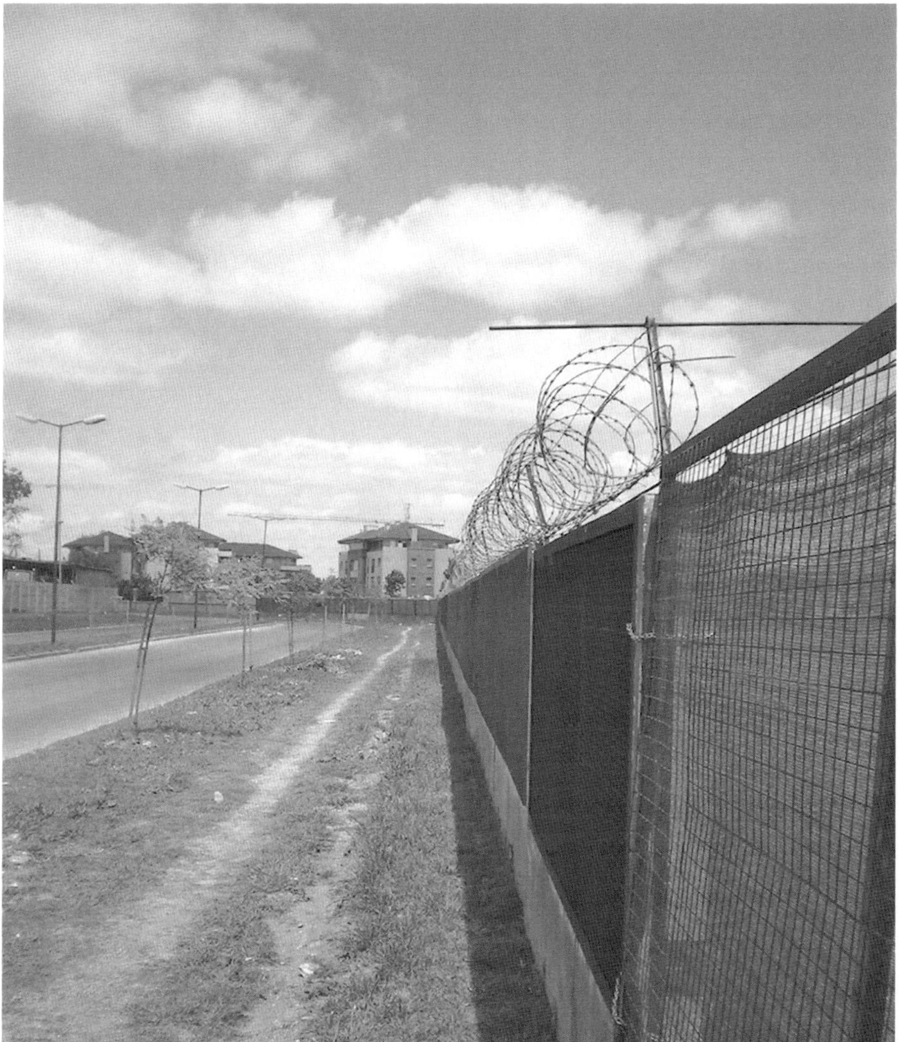

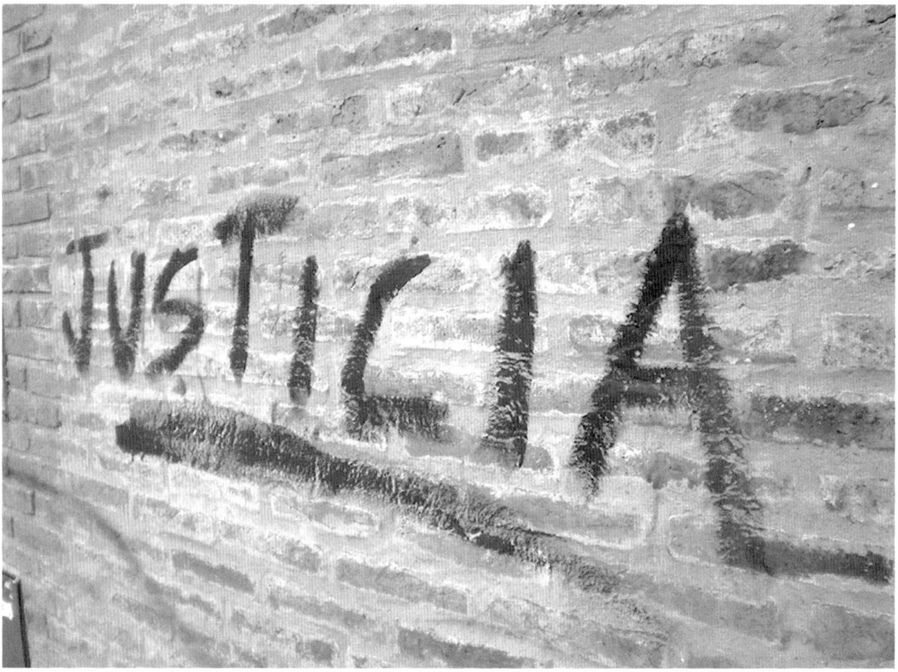
JUSTICIA

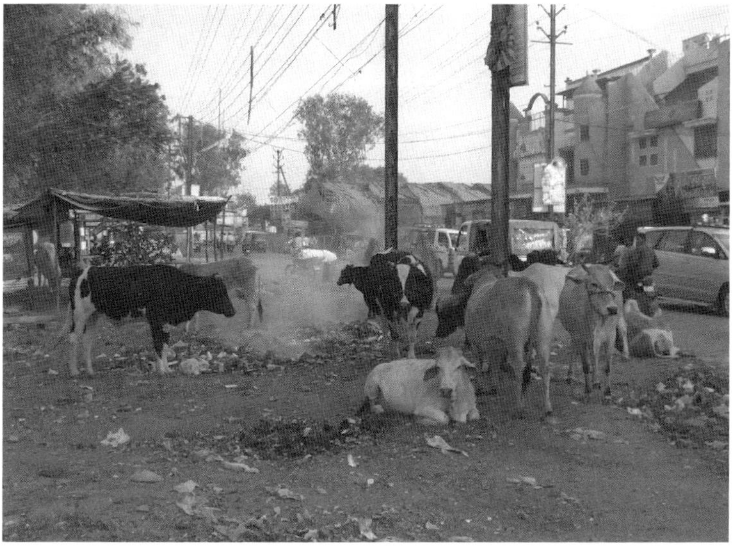

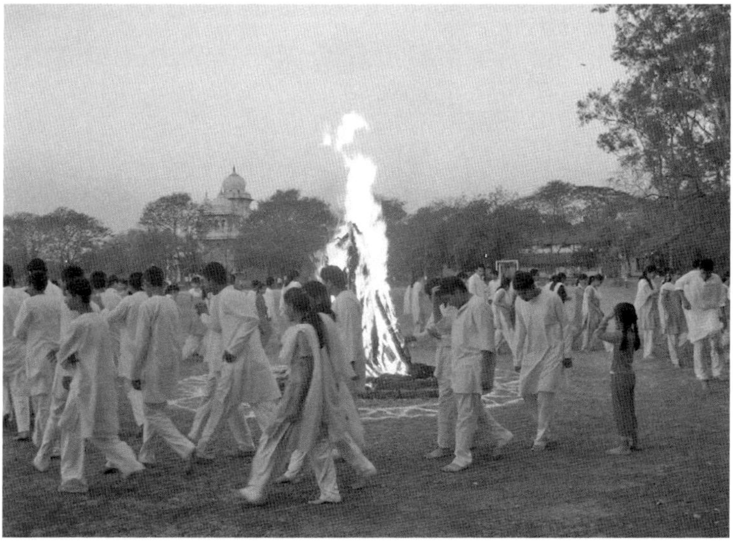

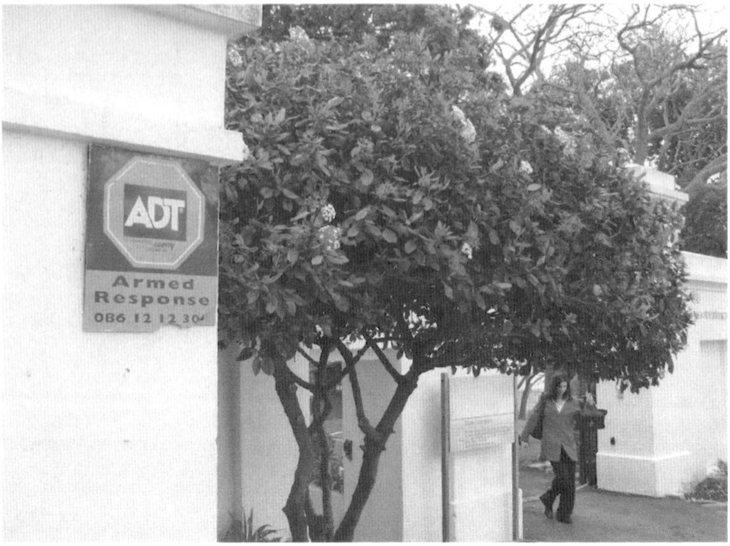

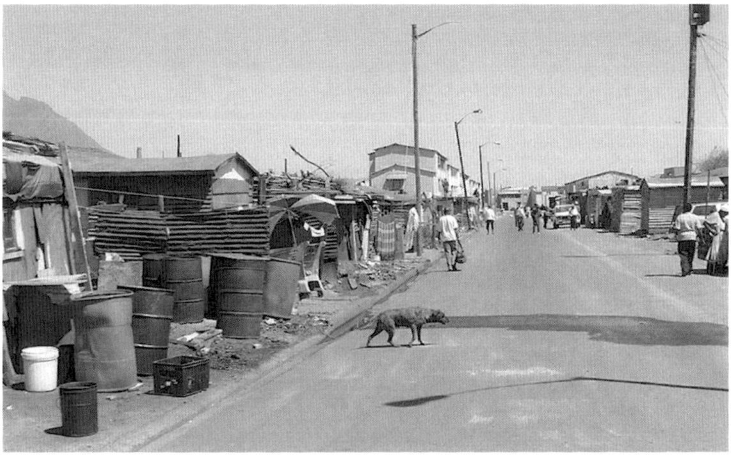

Photo courtesy of Chell Hill

Johannah Fahey is Senior Research Fellow in the Faculty of Education at Monash University, Australia. Her research interests are located in the areas of education and global studies, and are informed by her expertise in cultural studies. She has a national and international reputation in the areas of intersectionality (gender, race and class), and cultural globalization and mobilities. She is the co-editor of *Globalizing the Research Imagination* (Routledge 2009); and co-author/

author of *Haunting the Knowledge Economy* (Routledge 2006) and *David Noonan: Before and Now* (Thames and Hudson 2004). She has also published in many eminent international journals and edited books. She is the leading Research Fellow on the international team conducting the research project called *Elite independent schools in globalising circumstances: a multi-sited global ethnography.*

The (Semiotics of) Social Aesthetics in an Elite School in Singapore: An Ethnographic Study

Aaron Koh

Introduction

This chapter situates the methodological exploration of doing ethnography in an elite school in Singapore within a broader changing field of ethnography in the research landscape in contemporary times. While ethnography remains a venerable methodology, the staunch 'fetishisation of method' (Sweetman 2009, p. 492) is giving way to more inventive ways of conducting ethnography. Michael Burawoy et al. (2000), for example, developed 'global ethnography' to study how the local in a myriad of domains responds to the exacting forces of globalization; Dick et al. (2006) experimented with multimedia tools as their methodological instrument to study the production of scientific knowledge in an interactive science discovery center in Wales. Working with multimedia required them to explore multimodal ethnography.

More recently, Sarah Pink (2009, 2013) adds to the methodological repertoire of ethnography. Her foray into 'visual' and 'sensory' ethnography has provided fresh fodder for researchers to work with new media forms such as photography, video and web-based media where 'the visual' becomes composite data for analysis. Indeed contemporary ethnography can no longer rely on traditional ethnographic interviews and observations, and immersion in a static field-site for a sustained period of time as practiced by the Malinowski and Chicago school of ethnography (O'Reilly 2009). The availability of new technologies and theoretical apparatus is indeed changing and expanding the way contemporary ethnography is carried out.

This chapter draws inspiration from David MacDougall's (1999) landmark Doon School project. It considers the methodological contribution of 'social aesthetics' to ethnography with a view to critique it. As a point of departure, specific to the ethnographic fieldwork conducted in an elite school in Singapore, taken from the bigger 'Elite Independent Schools in globalizing circumstances: a multi-sited global eth-

A. Koh (✉)
Nanyang Technological University, Singapore, Singapore
e-mail: aaron.koh@nie.edu.sg

J. Fahey et al. (eds.), *In the Realm of the Senses,* Cultural Studies and Transdisciplinarity in Education, DOI 10.1007/978-981-287-350-7_5

nography' project, this chapter argues for a semiotic turn to ethnography. Informed by a theory of semiotics, it is argued that the visual saturation in the school warrants a closer examination of the semiosis in its visual-scape that also contributes to ethnographic knowing. The chapter introduces *semiotic ecology* as a new conceptual and methodological framework to think about epistemology, design and educational research that brings together the visual field, semiotics and contemporary ethnography.

The chapter is organized in the following directions. I begin with a review of David MacDougall's ethnographic work in the Doon School with the intention of fleshing out the contributions and limitations of 'social aesthetics'—a term he developed 'to invoke the sensorial, affective and aesthetic dimension of the lives and environments of the participants in (his) research' (Pink 2009, p. 139). This is followed up by a brief write-up of Straits School, the research context of the study. Next, I introduce *semiotic ecology* as a new epistemological and conceptual framework that contributes to the development of contemporary ethnography. I present some methodological issues specific to working with photographic images before offering a sampler analysis of the semiotic ecology in Straits School. The concluding section acknowledges some limitations of the study and synthesis of the ideological work of the semiotic ecology in the school.

The Methodological Benefits and Limitations of 'Social Aesthetics' for Ethnography

When David MacDougall conducted his fieldwork in The Doon School in India he expanded the epistemology and methodological design of doing ethnography. While still staying true to 'observation' as the essence of ethnography, he countered 'the hegemony of text' (O'Reilly 2009, p. 221) in ethnography by experimenting with film as a medium of representing the social and lifeworld of the school. It is to be noted that as a point of departure from the Malinowski tradition of doing ethnography, which essentially adheres to a realist frame of studying and interpreting culture in a field-site, MacDougall isolates the significance of the sensory and aesthetic environments. Here is where his contribution to contemporary ethnography lies.

To fully appreciate how MacDougall has shifted ethnography as a field, a brief context of his fieldwork is necessary. He gained access into an elite boarding school in Northern India called The Doon School with the intention of making a film which studied the cross-cultural contact and socialization in the school (MacDougall 1999). However, almost as if by chance, his attention shifted to the quotidian everyday lifeworld of the school making observations such as 'clothing, colors, timetables, eating implements, tones of voice, and characteristic gestures and postures' (MacDougall 1999, p. 4). Such ethnographic observations are, however, perceived through the senses.

The life-world of the school has a 'multimodal' dimension to it. Various 'modes' of representation like the sound, sight, movement, space and tactile dimensions are intrinsic to the social life of the school. But the potential of exploring the methodological benefits of multimodality and ethnography escapes MacDougall—a point I will return to when I consider the limitations of his work. Instead, MacDougall was very much influenced by the 'sensorial turn' (Howes 2003, p. xii) in anthropology. His ethnographic fieldwork in Doon School valorized the sensory experience. But this is not all there is to it in terms of his methodological innovation. He argued that the boarding school is 'a world in miniature' and has 'its own distinctive material signature' (Howes 2003, p. 4). It is this ethnographic observation of a rich tapestry of the materiality of the boarding school that led him to coin the term 'social aesthetics', where the sensory plays a significant part in constructing ethnographic knowledge.

A proper definition of what MacDougall means by 'social aesthetics' is in order. With reference to the Doon School, put simply, 'social aesthetics' refers to 'ethnographers' engagements with the sociality and materiality of research' (Pink 2009, p. 10). MacDougall likens 'the social aesthetics field' to Bourdieu's notion of habitus, which suggests that the dispositions, attitudes and values of the school are embodied and embedded within the social aesthetics field of the school. But the habitus is known, perceived and experienced through the senses. Where MacDougall has contributed to ethnography, particularly in school setting, is his departure from the classic observational approach to ethnography where the ethnographic instruments of observation, writing fieldnotes and interviews are relied on as sources of data for constructing ethnographic knowledge. Instead, through the medium of film, he interprets the culture of Doon School by drawing attention to the conjunction of a '…range of culturally patterned sensory experience' (1999, p. 5) *and* 'objects and actions' in the social aesthetics field of the school.

At this juncture, I want to flag the reach of 'social aesthetics'. In other words, much as MacDougall has expanded the methodological repertoire of doing ethnography, I argue that methodologically, 'social aesthetics' is useful to a point. In considering the specificities of the elite school in Singapore where ethnographic work was conducted, I take the advice of Gunther Kress (2011, p. 241) 'to recognize the boundaries within which one theory works well and the 'regions beyond' where a call on another theory and its methodology might be the better option'. I therefore introduce 'semiotic ecology' as a new conceptual framework. But more on this later. I shall proceed to offer a critique of MacDougall's work.

First and foremost, what I find conceptually inadequate about 'social aesthetics' is it does not provide the ethnographer/researcher with a critical vocabulary to interpret what is realized through the senses. In reference to the Doon School, MacDougall (1999, p. 14) could only identify 'a set of themes that seemed to provide conceptual keys to the school's aesthetic structures and their importance in the lives of the students'. He goes on to identify these themes as 'hierarchy and threats to personal identity'…clothing, eating, informal games, and organized sports'…the phenomenon of homesickness'…and 'certain classes of objects such as uniforms, the stainless still utensils…trophies and prizes of various kinds…' (MacDougall 1999) and etc.

While the sensorial experience is clearly invoked in the field work, in my opinion, his ethnographic study has not dug deeper into the *significance* of the sensory experience of the social aesthetics field of Doon School. In other words, while social aesthetics as a methodological lens unearths the invisible rituals and practices of the school, it does not work with an analytic toolkit that critically interprets the 'objects and actions' found within the social aesthetics field of the school. Here is where I argue 'social aesthetics' could benefit from a theory of semiotics. In fact, MacDougall (1999) himself acknowledged that 'to describe the social role of *aesthetics* properly (its phenomenological reality) we may need a 'language' close to the multidimensionality of the subject itself–that is, a language operating in visual, aural, verbal, temporal and even (through synaestetic association) tactile domains' (MacDougall 1999, p. 16). This language can be derived from the semiotic concept of 'mode', which Gunther Kress (2010, p. 79) defines as 'a socially shaped and culturally given semiotic resource for making meaning'.

More than just a language, in the economy of semiotics, modes is a meaning system used to represent and communicate meanings. Kress (2009) argues that modes perform specific semiotic work. As cultural resources, the attention to modes allows the ethnographer to ask a few important questions coalesced around:

> …meaning making; about agency of meaning-makers and the constant (re)constitution of identity in sign- and meaning-making; about the (social) constraints faced in making meaning; around social semiosis and knowledge; how 'knowledge' is produced and shaped and constituted distinctly in different modes; and by whom. (Kress 2011, p. 242)

I argue that this is the usefulness of a semiotic lens for ethnography. A theory of semiotics digs into the essence of meanings embodied in 'objects and actions' found within the habitus of a school as modes are expressions of cultural meanings. Let me analyze MacDougall's sensory perception of the social aesthetics in the Doon School through the semiotic lens of *modes*.

The social aesthetics in the Doon School draws attention to various elements such as 'the design of buildings and grounds, the use of clothing and colors, the rules of dormitory life, the organization of students' time, particular style of speech and gesture, and the many rituals of everyday life that accompany such activities as eating, school gatherings, and sport…' (MacDougall 1999, p. 5). But as a concept, social aesthetics has little analytical purchase; it does not account for the significance of the affordances and representational meanings of the social aesthetics in the school. It is through the semiotic concept of mode that meanings are derived. Here I am drawing on Kress' (2009, p. 66) notion of 'modal fixing', which is a useful way of considering *what* meanings and knowledge are produced through the choice of a mode. In other words, the decision of choosing a particular design for the buildings and grounds of the Doon School is not arbitrary; meanings are framed through choices of modes.

Secondly, I find it problematic that MacDougall should dismiss the centrality of the significance of signs in his sensorial interaction of the 'objects and actions' in the Doon School. It is also a contradiction that, while 'social aesthetics' acknowledges the materiality of things, it does not take a vested interest in 'the semiotic/cultural resources which are available for the realization/materialization of meaning as a motivated sign' (Kress 2010, p. 57). MacDougall comes close to valuing the importance of signs as semiotic affordances when he says that 'signs and meanings … clearly are at the school'. But the problem of signs for him is that they are overdetermined with meanings. There is also the propensity to yield to a decontextualized reading. In essence, his contention is that signs and their meanings are arbitrarily determined. Semioticians, however, reject such a view. Instead, they argue that all signs are motivated (Kress 2010); they are to be treated as 'semiotic inventories' (van Leeuwen, 2005, p. 6) assembled to communicate meanings. MacDougall's investment in the sensory experience, however, led him to privilege the 'sense impressions' (MacDougall 1999, p. 9) rather than the semiotic affordances of the materiality of social aesthetics.

As I evaluate the 'reach' of 'social aesthetics', in spite of its limitations, MacDougall is to be credited for his methodological contribution to ethnography, in particular, the sense perception of ethnographic knowing. His work has since been more substantially developed by Sarah Pink (2009) who named this expansion of ethnography as 'sensory ethnography'. Without going into the methodological details of what doing sensory ethnography entails, it suffices to mention briefly here that there is a more self-conscious and reflexive emphasis on the ethnographer's engagement with the senses throughout the research process (Pink 2009).

Yet in a more recent article, Pink (2011) examines the possibility of combining sensory ethnographic methodologies with multimodality. She pointed out that, despite coming from different theoretical premises and methodological approaches, contemporary ethnography can benefit from an assemblage of approaches. This seems to acknowledge that contemporary ethnography needs to call for new conceptual and methodological innovations while still working with classical approaches of doing ethnography. This chapter is positioned in the contemporary developments in ethnography. Specific to the elite school I was studying in Singapore, the classic observational approach of conducting ethnographic work was used with a view to understand the culture of the school, in tandem with a theory of social semiotics. I introduce the term 'semiotic ecology' to advance the epistemology and methodological design of doing ethnography. But, first, a brief contextual background on the school where the research was conducted.

Straits School: The Research Context

A premiere school in Singapore, Straits School has a long history that dates back to the colonial history of Singapore. Its exact founding was traced to 1823. As one of the oldest all boys' school in Singapore, the school has a legacy of producing many national leaders in every field although a concentration of political leaders herald from the school. The school is also noted internationally as the 'gateway to the Ivy Leagues' as it has produced the most number of students who successfully gained entry to the prestigious Oxbridge and Ivy League universities. The school's 2009/2010 annual report, for example, noted that over 335 students had secured places in Oxbridge and top US universities.

In the Singaporean landscape of schools, Straits School belongs to the league of independent schools, of which there are only eight. The school is also a boarding school and offers the Cambridge General Certificate Examination Advanced Level (GCE A Level) as the exit point in Year 12. It takes in boys only from Years 7 to 10 and becomes co-ed from Year 11 to 12. Unlike the majority of Singapore schools which offer the traditional academic pathway of the GCE O levels in Year 10, students in Straits School 'skip' the O levels as it is a school that offers the Integrated Program (IP), known also in local terms as 'through-train'. The IP is only meant for selected schools like Straits School which has a track record of outstanding achievements in academic and co-curricular activities. In replacement of the O levels, students in Straits School are afforded the opportunity to pursue an area of interest as part of their Gap Semester in Year 10.

Competition to get into the school is fierce. The school takes in 'the best of the best' (1–3 %) of high achievers determined by the Primary School Leaving Examination (PSLE) scores in Grade 6, although students with exceptional talents in Sports, Aesthetics and Arts are also considered for entry through the Direct School Admission (DSA). The school also takes in international students from the regions of China, Malaysia, Vietnam, Indonesia and others.

Straits School belongs to a network of international coalitions of elite schools, where there is a strong partnership in the domains of leadership education, pedagogy and teacher/student exchange programs. The school also has a strong culture of Service Learning where students are encouraged to perform community service in local communities and the wider region. On our first round of fieldwork in the school, we witnessed how the school was abuzz with calls for Service Learning as banners hung all over an empty area and along stairways in one of the teaching blocks. Indeed the school believes a good leader must begin with service. That is why it gives undue emphasis to Service Learning.

Semiotic Ecology: An Epistemological and Conceptual Framework

In this part of the chapter, I make constant reference to the exclusive 'we' because Jane Kenway and I teamed up as a pair of 'insider-outsider' ethnographer in Straits School in May 2011 for 3 weeks in the school to collect data. As a Singaporean who had been through Singapore's education system first as a student, then a teacher, and now a researcher, I am the insider who possess the knowledge of the cultural context of the fieldsite, whereas Jane is the outsider looking in, also playing the role of making the familiar strange for me. This synergistic 'insider-outsider' teamwork benefits the ethnographic fieldwork in the school as we co-constructed ethnographic knowledge of the school with perspectives that did not always agree, and for good reasons.

However, what we agreed on, almost without debate, was the rich saturation of semiotic artefacts (such as banners, photographs, flyers from clubs and societies, objects, artwork, and even the architecture of buildings) that filled every space and corner of the school that we thought were important visual data, in addition to the traditional ethnographic interviews and observations we were collecting. The various buildings in the school such as school hall, boarding school, admin block, the school library, and etc. too caught our attention because these various buildings were themselves a visual spectacle. Collectively these semiotic artefacts and displays jumped at us like 'floating signifiers' waiting for us to decode their meanings. We also began to question the ideological work they do.

Almost instinctively, we knew we had to collect all these 'semiotic inventories' (van Leeuwen 2005, p. 6) by using our digital cameras. I shall explain the process of collecting visual data in a later section under methodology. Indeed the 'semiotic excess' in the school compound demanded our ethnographic attention and called for analytic work around the school's semiotic ecology—a term that befits the visual saturation in the school. But there is more to semiotic ecology as a descriptor. It was after the fieldwork that I began conceptualizing the term as a way of framing our visual data theoretically and analytically driven by a theory of social semiotics.

'Ecology' is defined in dictionaries and its derivative in research is used rather consistently. Most dictionaries (see for example Collins Cobuild) emphasize the intricate relationship between people, plants, animals and their environment. In sociolinguistics, ecology is used as a metaphor to refer to 'the study of interaction between any given language and its environment' (Haugen 2001, p. 57). This metaphor suggests that there is a functional link between language and its environment. Research in new media and young people has also latched on to the *ecology* metaphor coining the term 'media ecology' to describe the 'changing and variegated set of media ecologies' in which young people participate (Ito et al. 2009, p. 30). Here the ecology metaphor is used to indicate that new media has become a part of young peoples' lives. The concepts of 'system' and 'equilibrium' are also crucial in ecology—whether the ecological sciences or ecology as used in social science, say, urban ecology (the Chicago school of urban studies in the early twentieth century) (Gottdiener and Budd 2005).

Not unlike how ecology is used in the above, I am using 'semiotic ecology' to describe the richly textual, material, and multimodal visual-scape of the school, all of which are treated as 'semiotic resources'. Following Theo van Leeuwen (2005, p. 3), I am using 'semiotic resource/s' here—a key term in social semiotics—to refer to 'the actions and artefacts we use to communicate (meanings)…'. Inherent in all semiotic resources is the assumption that they contain 'semiotic potentials' (van Leeuwen 2005, p. 4) for making meaning. But these meanings are contextually derived rather than arbitrarily determined.

I further use 'semiotic ecology' to suggest that all the sedimented semiotic resources found in the school contribute to the sum effect of what Scollon and Scollon (2003, p. 175) call 'semiotic aggregate'. That is to say all the semiotic resources add up, interact and converge in the ecology of the school to form a composite meaning, which can be read off, and also tell us about the impression management of Straits School. The school, and all the semiotic resources contained within are therefore treated as a huge semiotic structure. This term therefore advances the epistemology of ethnography arguing that ethnographic knowing does not reside in interviews and what MacDougall (1999) has called sensory ethnography. Rather, I argue for a semiotic turn in the methodological repertoire of doing ethnography where a foray into the semiotic affordances of the ecology of the school can contribute to the ethnographic knowledge.

Importantly, my intention of using the ecology metaphor is to foreground the symbiotic links between the disparate semiotic elements found in the school and the wider ecological geography of the school. Bearing in mind the salience of 'system' and 'equilibrium' central in ecology, my analysis of the semiotic ecology in Straits School will suggest that the re/production of privilege, power and prestige is the overriding logic that organizes its semiotic ecology. As my analysis of the representative visual data collected later will reveal, the semiotic inventories gathered function as impression management at one level, and for ideological posturing at another level. However, because the metaphor of 'ecology' is essentially a place-based system, any attempts to decode the visual ideology embodied by the semiotic ecology in the school must be situated in the wider context of the socio-cultural and histories of the school.

The Contributions of 'Semiotic Ecology' for Ethnography

What, then, are the benefits of semiotic ecology for ethnography? Firstly, it treats the visual-scape of the school as a system of representation that communicates meanings—meanings that point to specific construction of the ethos, values and culture of the school, what might also be called the social imagination of the school. However, this ideological level of meaning may not be immediately transparent for the analyst/viewer because ideologies are often 'buried'. They appear to be natural or given and their meanings camouflaged as denotations (Sturken and Cartwright 2001). It must also be said that the aesthetic and emotive appeal of visuals often occlude the more important ideological meanings. A semiotic ethnographic lens therefore invites us to 'study the hidden meanings' (Harper 2012, p. 118)—the ideological meanings that are embedded in all artefacts, buildings and architectural designs, and things 'visual' used as 'semiotic aggregates' (Scollon and Scollon 2003, p. 175) to *position* the school in a certain light. Such an inquiry opens up the knowledge construction in ethnographic fieldwork where social semiosis is a source of contribution (Kress 2011).

Secondly, as an epistemological design, 'semiotic ecology' also provides the toolkit to dig into the 'appearances' of the visual-scape in the school. Here I shall take a short excursion to explain two core concepts in semiotic theory, which is central as 'tools' for analysis in a later section.

In the economy of semiotics, inherent in the semiological system are two levels of meanings, one denotative and the other, connotative. Denotative meanings are derived from 'the use of semiotic resources that refer to concrete people, places, things, qualities and events' (van Leeuwen 2005, p. 275). In other words, there is a direct correspondence between the object referred to and resource used. Call it the first layer of meaning if you like, denotative meaning essentially asks the question 'what, or who, is represented here?' (van Leeuwen 2005, p. 37). It is also at the denotative level of meaning that I suggest emotive appeal and aesthetic beauty of visual exemplars are appreciated.

Connotative meanings, on the other hand, is the second layer of the meaning superimposed on denotative meaning, derived from '*culturally shared associations* which cling to the represented people, places and things, or through specific 'connotators'…' (van Leeuwen 2005, p. 38; my emphasis). It is also at this level that ideological meanings reside. It is important to note, however, that because connotative meanings rely on 'culturally shared associations', it is not often that this level of meaning is realized because the viewer may not possess the culture-specific knowledge. Meaning-making therefore may be reduced to guess work. However, there are semiotic resources intrinsic in the semiological system that functions as 'connotators' that unlock this level of meaning; for example, how the represented object poses, the specific style and techniques used to enhance the visual object are examples of 'connotators' (van Leeuwen 2005, p. 39). These 'connotators' are by themselves layered with semiotic affordances contributing to the ideological meanings.

In sum, the benefits of 'semiotic ecology' as an epistemological and conceptual framework are: it draws critical attention to ideological representation of the visual-scape of the school, at the same time provides the analytical vocabularies for the ethnographer to unpack the ideological work of the semiotic affordances in the ecology of the school.

Researching 'Lived Visual Data': Methodological Issues

In addition to taking field-notes and interviewing, as part of our immersion in the school we took photographs of the striking semiotic ecology. Jane and I became 'visualista' (Spencer 2011, p. 1)—a term used by Eric Margolis to name visual researchers. We walked around the school campus (which is roughly the size of 12 football fields) and took photographs of the things we 'see' and 'sense' as important for our ethnographic study of the school.

Broadly, the methodology used in this study is distilled from an emerging methodological field called 'visual research method' (Rose 2011, 2013). As ethnographers in the school, our methodological commitment was to enlist a 'research method' that would help us gather a 'thick description' of the school in more ways than one. A methodological clarification is, however, needed here. While we actively sought out to collect images in the semiotic ecology of the school, we were less concerned with what meanings were inherent in the photographs. Rather, we were more concern with what using 'visual research method' was able to help us achieve (Rose 2013).

Taking photographs was the methodological instrument for us as researchers to 'store' and revisit the sights and perceptions of the school. Methodologically, it was important for us to do this because on one hand, we wanted to capture our dwelling in the school as ethnographers and turned the semiotic ecology into 'lived visual data' (Emerson et al. 2013, p. 5). This term suggests that we captured our sight of the semiotic inventories in the school and turned them into 'a form of 'lived text', where a visual bank of the semiotic ecology of Straits School can be further analyzed to reveal the hidden cultural values and norms (Emmison 2013, p. 5).

On the other hand, we also noted how some of the visual exemplars in the ecology were not permanent fixtures. Over the 3-year sequential visits to the school from 2011 to 2013, we noticed that some of the visual artefacts we saw in year 1 of our visit no longer existed upon our second visit in the subsequent year, while others remain. Yet new ones emerged in year 3 of our fieldwork. Had we not taken photographs in the first round of our ethnographic work, we would not be able to account for the fluidity and dynamics of the semiotic ecology of the school. One such ephemeral semiotic exemplar (see Fig. 3) is analyzed in the section below as a case in point.

In the literature on visual research methods, Gillian Rose pointed out that there is a tendency for visual researchers to 'focus on the *visibility* rather than *visuality*' (Rose 2013, p. 9; emphasis original) of their research. That is to say visual researchers tended to use photographs to show, making things visible instead of viewing visual data 'as meaning objects central to symbolic and communicative activity' (Rose 2013, p. 9). This study attempts to do both. It uses photographic images to document and create an archive of images to make explicit the *visibility* of the social life of the school. The conceptual framing of the semiotic ecology of the school as elaborated above, however, was developed to foreground and analyzed the school's *visuality*.

Before I proceed to offer and analyze a sampler of the visibility and visuality of the semiotic ecology in Straits School as 'lived visual data', it is important that I mention some ethical considerations and challenges related to the visual methodology of this study.

Emmison et al. (2013, p. 8) mentioned that 'the act of seeing comes with responsibilities'. I want to further suggest that in addition to seeking consent from the institutions concerned to take photographs of the research site, our 'ethical' responsibilities further require us to practice auto-self censorship. For instance, when choosing images for public presentation, we doctored some images to conceal the identity of the school whilst others that were too upfront remain as archival materials in our restricted confluence website. The extent to which we observed the ethics of working with images is because we had to be sensitive to the social, cultural and political context of Singapore, particularly at a time where the politics of privilege and elitism in its education landscape and wider social domain remain contentious and sensitive issues (see Koh 2014).

However, we found it a challenge to hide the identity of the school because Singapore is a small country. It does not help that the school we were researching has an international reputation. When we presented our papers from the project overseas at international conferences, our audience could second guess which elite schools were our fieldsites. Bound by ethics of research, we remain tight-lip however. Our refrain has been 'you can guess but we can't confirm'. Clearly for our research team, working with images on elite schools is a methodological dilemma.

Semiotic Ecology in Straits School: A Sampler Analysis

In the sampler photo images that I have selected for analysis in this chapter, each photo is given a caption. This is to counter the polysemic affordances of a visual image. The caption is, however, not randomly chosen. It is derived from the emic perspective of the researcher. The theoretical premise of 'semiotic ecology' also argues for a strong contextual knowledge to arrive at the connotative level of meaning (Harper 2012). Without providing an anchor to the photo images, the meaning/s of the image will remain unstable, open to an array of interpretations.

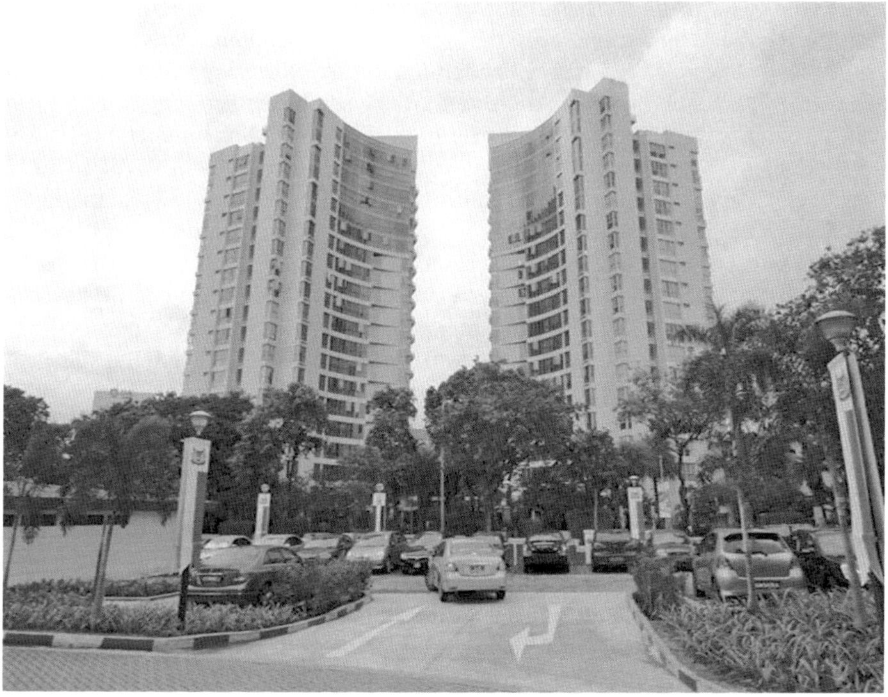

Fig. 1 Elite Association

The meaning of this photo image appears somewhat transparent, at least at the denotative level (See Fig. 1). This is because the indexicality of the photo immediately connects the viewer to two high rise apartments facing directly opposite the main entrance of the school. In a sense then, this image presents an apparently unarguable reality—it tells us in no uncertain terms that it is the main entrance of a place even if no insider contextual knowledge is provided. But there is more to the meaning of the photo image.

This photo was taken and included as a significant semiotic inventory in the semiotic ecology of the school because the two apartments bear some relationship to the school although only in name. I took this photo because the condominiums carry the name of the school. It is called 'Straits Condo'. For 'outsiders', it can easily be mistaken that the condominiums are properties of the school, perhaps used as staff quarters. This is where I argue the semiosis of the photo image depends on the cultural knowledge of the fieldsite. This in turn has significant bearings on the connotative meaning and the overall semiotic aggregate meaning of the visual-scape of the school.

'Straits Condo' was built in 2002 on a prime location mainly because it is directly opposite Straits School and located conveniently within walking distance to two rail stations (i.e. known locally as MRT) and a shopping mall. A check on the internet of the valuation price of this landed property reveals that it is valued in the range of SGD1.2 m to SGD1.5 million in the Singapore property market. Here a further socio-cultural understanding of the significance of condominiums as 'symbolic goods' is necessary. In Singapore condominiums are expensive private properties afforded by the upper middle class and above, whereas the majority of Singaporeans reside in government built high-rise flats, also known locally as HDB flats. In local popular discourse, condominiums are often said to be one of the 5Cs (Cash, Car, Credit Cards, Country Club memberships) that constitutes the materiality of the 'Singaporean dream'.

The connotative meaning of this photo resides in the association of 'Straits Condo' to Straits School. That a landed property has taken the name of a school signifies that 'Straits' has been turned into a 'brand' name. As a brand name, Straits has become a sign in the semiological system that connotes the symbolic values of prestige, social standing, class and power. As explained, condominiums are *exclusive* housing in Singapore. By association, Straits is also an exclusive elite school. The name of the school has such commanding power that it has not only elevated the value of property prices in the vicinity, but also invited investors to build properties such as 'Straits Condo', clearly capitalizing on the prestige of the school Fig. 2 (i.e. the photo) here.

This gallery of photos depicts famous alumni that Straits School has produced. In our three rounds of ethnographic work in the school over three consecutive years, this semiotic inventory remains a permanent fixture in the semiotic ecology of the school, and for good reasons. The denotative meaning of the photos is striking enough to catch the viewer's attention. This is because the photographs index real people and significantly, these 'real people' are politicians in Singapore from different generations. Of course, such revelation requires the viewer to have contextual knowledge of the photographs, and in this case, the 'who's who' in the political arena of Singapore.

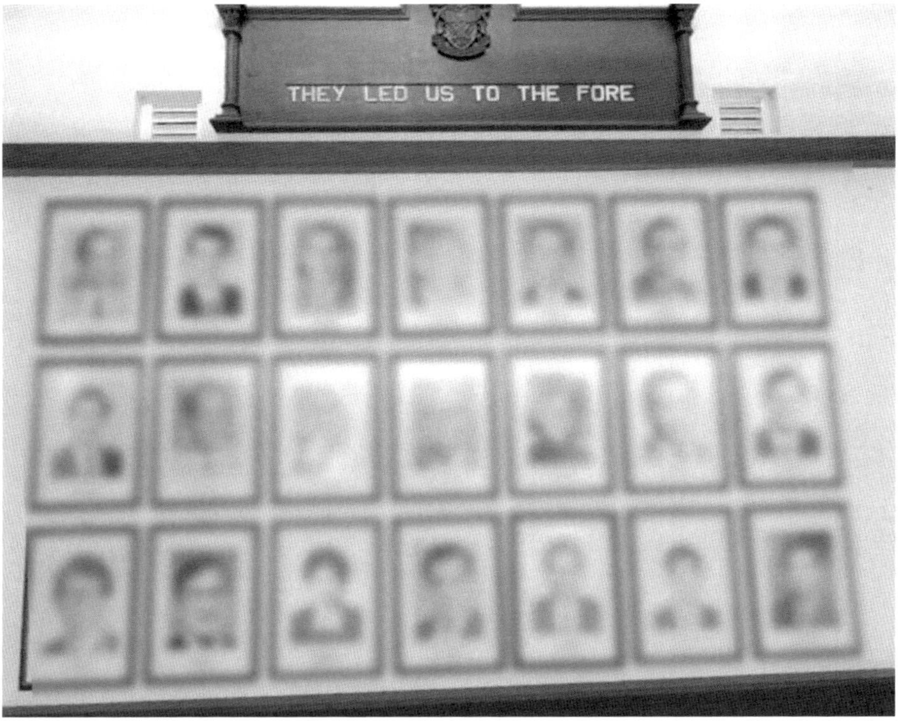

Fig. 2 Hall of Fame

But even without the emic perspective, there are specific 'connotators' (van Leeuwen 2005) from the photo images that indicate that the people in the photographs are important people; for example, the framing is a close-up indicating their stature; the black and white photographs conveys that the school has a legendary history of producing power elites, and the formal wear connotes power and status. The frontal angle of the photographs and the 'visual demand' (Kress and van Leeuwen 2006, p. 118) defined as the imaginary friendly gaze emanating from the photograph that connects the viewer, invite students of Straits to look up to them as role models because the linguistic text 'they led us to the fore' frames the meaning of the gallery of photos at the ideological level.

In the economy of semiotics, these 'connotators' are semiotic codes that work at an ideological level to communicate meanings. At one level, these photo images point to famous alumni at the denotative level. However, at another level, the linguistic text also turns the photo images into iconic signs, at the same time infused the gallery of photos with symbolic meanings. This is an example of the complex work of a sign that condenses the layers of meanings into an entity. Straits School is an *iconic* elite school in Singapore in part because of the association of the ranks of these famous alumni that the school has produced. They thus operate as *symbols* of achievement that the school has come to be known for. But importantly, the display functions ideologically as 'models of inspiration' for students.

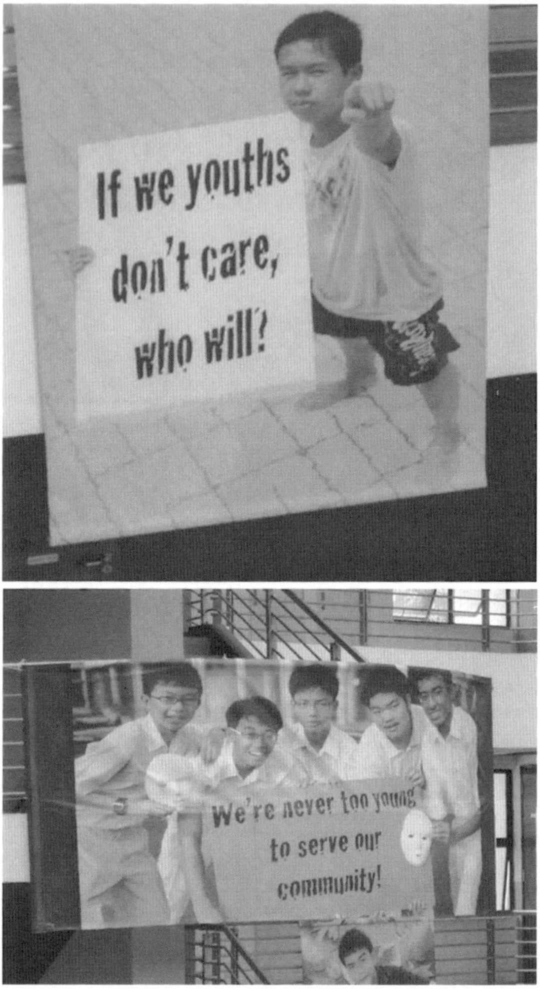

Fig. 3 Service learning banners

We saw a series of such banners advocating Service Learning in a classroom block in the first round of fieldwork. These banners were no longer a part of the semiotic ecology of the school when we returned a year later. Figure 3 is therefore an example of an ephemeral semiotic exemplar.

At the denotative level, these banners were created with a specific audience in mind: encouraging the wider student community in Straits to take part in Service Learning. There is a specific 'visual grammar' (Kress and van Leeuwen 2006) shared by the two banners. Both photographs perform a 'visual demand' although the gaze in Fig. 3a is more commanding as the represented participant points his finger at the viewer. The authoritative tone of the photo image is reinforced by the linguistic text 'if we youths don't care, who will!'. The smiling faces of Fig. 3b on the other hand invites the viewer to enter into a social affinity with them as their smiles seem to suggest they derive pleasure and satisfaction from service.

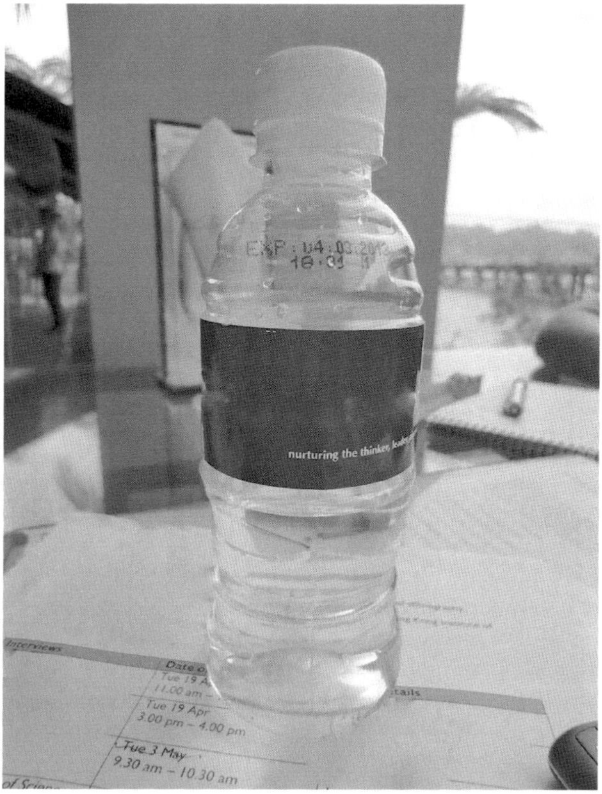

Fig. 4 'Corporate' Straits School

In all, the 'connotators' in the two images carry the themed message of participating in Service Learning, but one targets an apathetic group of students (i.e. Fig. 3a) who either are disinterested or simply do not care, while the other (i.e. Fig. 3b) solicits participation with a more inclusive and congenial message of 'we're never too young to serve our community'.

But this is not all the meanings of the photo image. There is a hidden, ideological meaning which remains buried unless a contextual knowledge of the school culture is given. There is a strong narrative and cultivation of service as an important ethos in Straits School. The school management believes that as part of leadership cultivation it is important that students learn to serve before they can lead. Learning to serve also keeps students who come from more privilege backgrounds aware of the reality of the existence of the less fortunate around them. Therefore, at an ideological level, this photo image while advocating service learning also conceals that service learning is a disciplinary project that aims to foster in students the values of humility and empathy. Read ideologically, Service Learning also functions as a disavowal practice as the school wards of suggestions of privilege and elitism that it has come to be associated with.

This photo image indexes a bottle of mineral water (Fig. 4). We thought this semiotic artefact was an important semiotic inventory because not all schools in

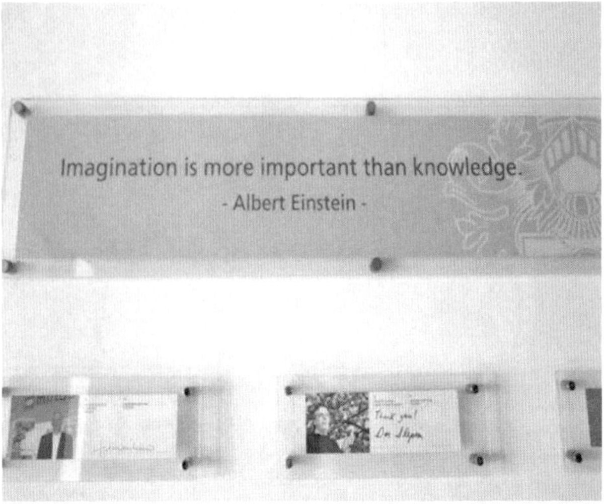

Fig. 5 Elite 'connections'

Singapore provides their guests with the school's own brand of mineral water. The denotative reference while obvious, however, sheds its ordinariness because the bottle of mineral water has undergone semiotic change clearly marked as a complex sign with semiotic codes like the school color, crest, logo and credo. These are, however, not readable from the photo image because it has been 'photoshopped' to conceal the identity of the school.

This branded bottle of mineral water has a new social biography (cf. Appadurai 1988). From an ordinary mineral water bottle, the now *branded* bottle connotes ideas of corporatization as well as branding that have become a significant aspect of the impression management of the school. This semiotic artefact is an indication that the school has embraced corporatization, where branding is mobilized in the representation of the school. However, unlike 'branding' which is widely used to launch a new product and to increase sales, 'branding' is used in the school strategically to project a public image of the quality of education that Straits offers. This is the ideological meaning, also realized at the connotative meaning of the mineral water bottle (Fig. 4).

We took photographs of these images on a wall in the new school building because the narrative seems strikingly obvious (see Fig. 5). These semiotic artefacts serve as a visual record of famous people who have visited the school. However, it is not clear at the denotative level of meaning whether the visitors were invited by the school or they visited the school on their own accord. But what is made abundantly clear is: the visitors are in a league of their own. From their institution affiliations and titles, we know these visitors are either famous professors hailing from elite universities such as Cambridge, Oxford, London School of Economics, and national leaders. Thus, what we can see from the gallery of images are 'impressions' of real people whom we are unlikely to know or remember, but their institutional affiliations and titles register an immediate connection because these are world famous universities.

However, it is the level of connotation that powerfully suggests the significance of the associations of these 'royal' visits. It is unlikely that these visitors would fly all the way to Singapore just to visit Straits School if it was not for its international reputation. In other words, by association, these visual records of their visit connote that Straits School is an iconic elite school that has a global standing. This gallery of photo images also serves to showcase the strong international/global network that the school has become a part of. Indeed, the name and repute of the school has travelled. People are visiting Straits because it is an exceptional school.

Conclusion

Concluding the chapter with a final commentary I ask, from the analysis presented above, what is the 'semiotic aggregate' of these representative semiotic inventories in the semiotic ecology of Straits School and what is the overall 'system' and 'equilibrium' in the semiotic ecology striving for?

In this chapter, my intent has been to contribute to contemporary ethnography by drawing on a theory inspired methodology that draws on semiotics to analyze ethnographic visual data. Recall that 'semiotic ecology' is a conceptual framework mobilized to harness together the semiosis that goes on in the visual-scape in the school, it also observes a symbiosis between the semiotic resources found in the school and its embedded ecology. While each of the semiotic inventories produces layers of meaning, the composite meaning of all the semiotic exemplars add up to produce a 'semiotic aggregate' about the ideological work of the semiosis that takes place in the ecology.

To synthesize my analysis, outside the school, the name of condominiums by association with the school takes on the symbolic values of prestige and class. Within the school, the elite identity of the school is further reinforced by photo images in the 'Hall of Fame' that portray a stellar cast of national leaders as 'models of inspiration' for the students. As an iconic elite school, whose repute has travelled, the school has invited 'elite arrivals' and forged 'connections' at various levels. It becomes necessary for the school to present a corporatized image to the public embodied by the branded mineral water bottle.

Yet Service Learning is steeped in the culture of the school mobilized as a form of disciplinary apparatus to cultivate the values of humility and empathy in students. Seen from a larger ideological perspective, Service Learning functions as a disavowal practice of the school to defray criticisms of elitism and privilege often levelled at elite schools. Clearly, the semiotic ecology of the school performs the ideological work of posturing and (elite) identity management, mirroring to the school population and the wider public how it likes to be seen and known. Overall, 'privilege', 'power' and 'prestige' yet a school that reaches out to the less privilege in the wider communities are the organizing 'systems' and 'equilibrium' the semiotic ecology of the school is striving for.

Finally, while this chapter has illustrated the methodological benefits of semiotics to examine the visual-scape in an elite school, there is definitely scope for the further development of semiotic inspired ethnography drawing on an assemblage of theories and analytical tools.

References

Appadurai, A. (Ed.). (1988). *The social life of things: Commodities in cultural perspective*. Cambridge: Cambridge University Press.

Burawoy, M., Blum, J. A., George, S., Gille, Z., & Thayer, M. (2000). *Global Ethnography: Forces, connections and imaginations in a postmodern world*. Berkeley: University of California Press.

Dicks, B., Soyinka, B., & Coffey, A. (2006). Multimodal ethnography. *Qualitative Research, 6*(1), 77–96.

Emmison, M., Smith, P., & Mayall, M. (2013). *Researching the visual* (2nd ed.). London: Sage.

Gottdiener, M., & Budd, L. (2005). *Key concepts in urban studies*. London: Sage.

Harper, D. (2012). *Visual sociology*. London: Routledge.

Haugen, E. (2001). The ecology of language. In A. Fill & P. Muhlhauster (Eds.), *The ecolinguistics reader: Language, ecology and environment* (pp. 57–66). London: Continuum.

Howes, D. (2003). *Sensual relations: Engaging the senses in culture and social theory*. Ann Arbor: The University of Michigan Press.

Ito, M., Horst, H., Bittanti, M., Boyd, D., Herr-Steohenson, B., Lange, P., Pascoe, C., & Robinson, L. (2009). *Living and learning with new media: Summary of findings from the Digital Youth Project*. The John D. and Catherine T. MacArthur Foundation reports on digital media and learning. Cambridge: The MIT Press.

Koh, A. (2014). Doing class analysis in Singapore's elite education: Unravelling the smokescreen of 'meritocratic talk'. *Globalisation, Societies & Education, 2*(1). (in press).

Kress, G. (2009). What is mode? In C. Jewitt (Ed.), The Routledge handbook of multimodaly analysis (pp. 54–67). London: Routledge.

Kress, G. (2010). *Multimodality: A social semiotic approach to contemporary communication*. London: Routledge.

Kress, G. (2011). 'Partnerships in research': Multimodality and ethnography. *Qualitative Research, 11*(3), 239–260.

Kress, G., & van Leeuwen, T. (2006). *Reading images: The grammar of visual design*. London: Sage.

MacDougall, D. (1999). Social aesthetics and the Doon School. *Visual Anthropology, 15*(1), 3–20.

O'Reilly, K. (2009). *Key concepts in ethnography*. London: Sage.

Pink, S. (2009). *Doing sensory ethnography*. London: Sage.

Pink, S. (2011). Multimodality, multsensoriality and ethnographic knowing: Social semiotics and the phenomenology of perception. *Qualitative Research, 11*(3), 261–276.

Pink, S. (2013). *Doing visual ethnography* (3rd ed.). London: Sage.

Rose, G. (2011). *Visual methodologies: Interpretating visual materials* (3rd ed.). London: Sage.

Rose, G. (2013). On the relation between 'visual research methods' and contemporary visual culture. *The Sociological Review,* 1–13. doi:10.1111/1467-954X.12109.

Scollon, R., & Scollon, S. W. (2003). *Discourse in place: Language in the material world*. London: Routledge.

Spencer, S. (2011). *Visual research methods in the social science: Awakening visions*. London: Routledge.

Sturken, M., & Cartwright, L. (2001). *Practices of looking: An introduction to visual culture*. Oxford: Oxford University Press.
Sweetman, P. (2009). Revealing habitus, illuminating practice: Bourdieu, photography and visual methods. *The Sociological Review, 57*(3), 493–511.
Van Leeuwen, T. (2005). *Introducing social semiotics*. London: Routledge.

Dr. Aaron Koh is Associate Professor, at the National Institute of Education, Singapore. His research areas are: Language Arts/Literacy, Cultural Studies in Education and Global Studies in Education. He is on the Editorial Board of *Curriculum Inquiry, Journal of Curriculum and Pedagogy, Discourse: studies in the cultural politics of education and Journal of Adolescent & Adult Literacy*. The politics at work in the local where government bodies mediate, interrupt and disrupt global forces for local conditions. While his context of analysis is primarily Singapore, he distils the theoretical frame borrowed from cultural studies to examine the relation between globalization and education in the East. He has contributed to this field by developing a multi-modal analytical approach to education policy analysis. He has published in many reputable international journals, edited several special issue journals and contributed a growing number of book chapters. His most recent book is Tactical Globalisation, (Peter Lang 2010).

Visual Essay: Semiotic Ecology

Johannah Fahey

Shifting Signs and Symbols of Privilege

Marble busts of Queen Victoria and a founding father on display in the corridors of Highbury Hall and Ripon College respectively harkens back to the height of Empire. They are emblematic of these elite schools affiliation with royalty and a sense of importance. And yet, Empire was not necessarily installed in the colonies without conflict, indeed these power struggles from the past are attested to in the present by the positioning of Macaulay's speech of 1835—where he speaks of the desire for India to become 'a truly dominated nation'—outside the school principal's office. Oil paintings of the school's original donors hang in gilded frames—that recall the European galleries of old—in a recently recreated darbar, and so the symbolic court of Indian princes nowadays holds images of Indian royalty that were painted by a renowned English portrait artist. The glory of these Raj princes in the early twentieth century has faded but is not forgotten as the skins of big cats exhibited in the school library uphold the hunting prowess of this privileged warrior caste. The lion, another big cat, a continuing symbol of not just strength and leadership, but the endurance of empire, remains emblazoned on the Founder's blazer, while the chimerical quality of the gryphon, half lion and half eagle, symbolizes the combined strength of colony and Empire at Straits School in Singapore. The far-sightedness associated with the eagle is manifest at Old Cloisters as aspiration: the Barbadian scholars boards are placed strategically above the heads and in full sight of the students when they assemble in the school hall. At Highbury Hall, it is the school 'leavers' that lead the way as a word cloud gives greater prominence to Oxbridge and we enter the realm of the elite university; while a cabinet of trophies adorns the entrance of Cathedral College's assembly hall, with the words 'Justice' and 'Honour' symbolically written above the threshold into the world beyond.

J. Fahey (✉)
Monash University, Melbourne, Australia
e-mail: johannah.fahey@monash.edu

J. Fahey et al. (eds.), *In the Realm of the Senses,* Cultural Studies and Transdisciplinarity in Education, DOI 10.1007/978-981-287-350-7_6

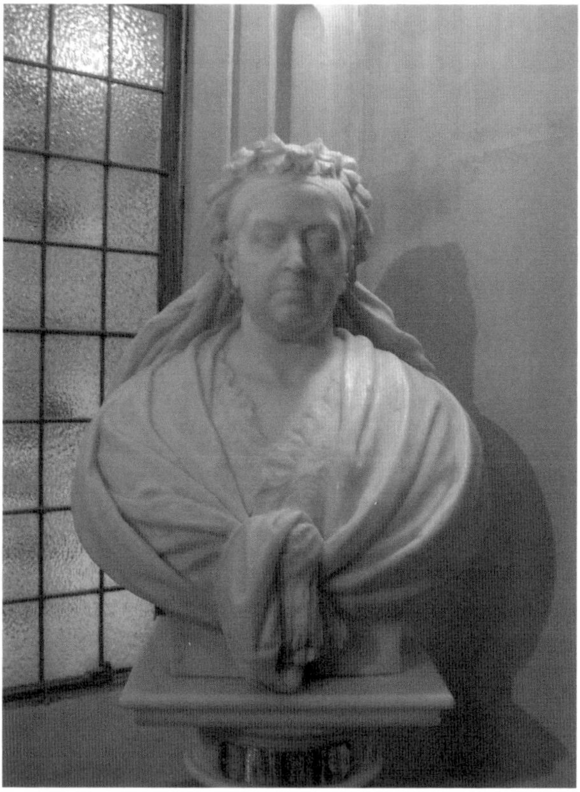

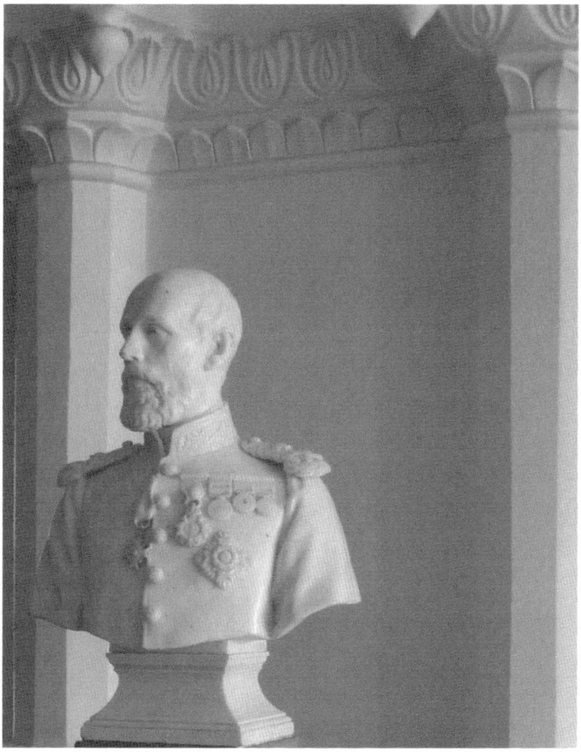

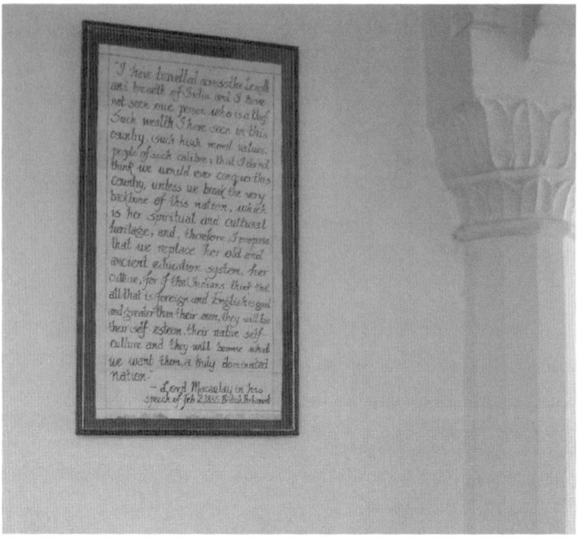
"I have travelled across the length and breadth of India and I have not seen one person who is a thief. Such wealth I have seen in this country, such high moral values, people of such calibre, that I do not think we would ever conquer this country, unless we break the very backbone of this nation, which is her spiritual and cultural heritage, and, therefore, I propose that we replace her old and ancient education system, her culture, for if the Indians think that all that is foreign and English is good and greater than their own, they will lose their self-esteem, their native self-culture and they will become what we want them, a truly dominated nation."
– Lord Macaulay in his speech of Feb 2 1835 British Parliament

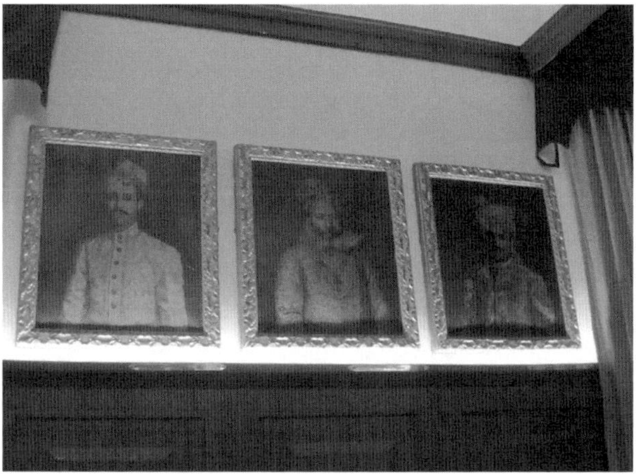

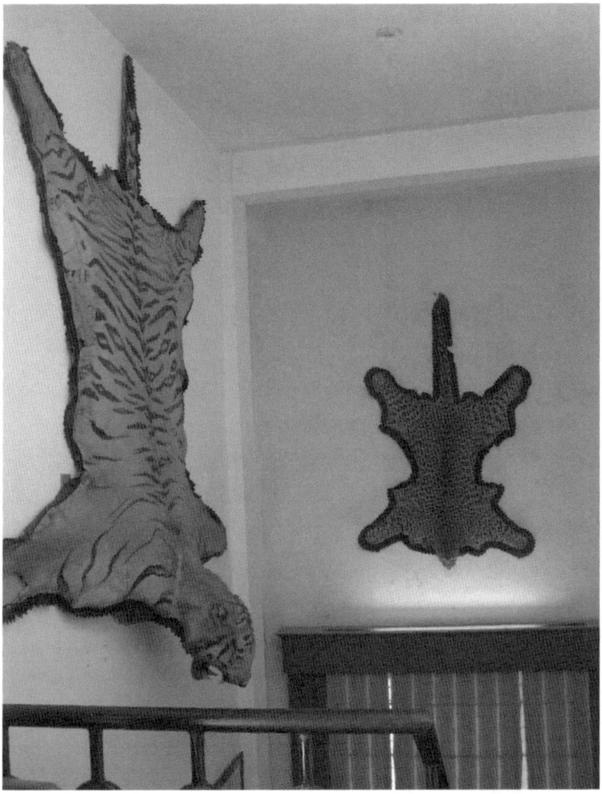

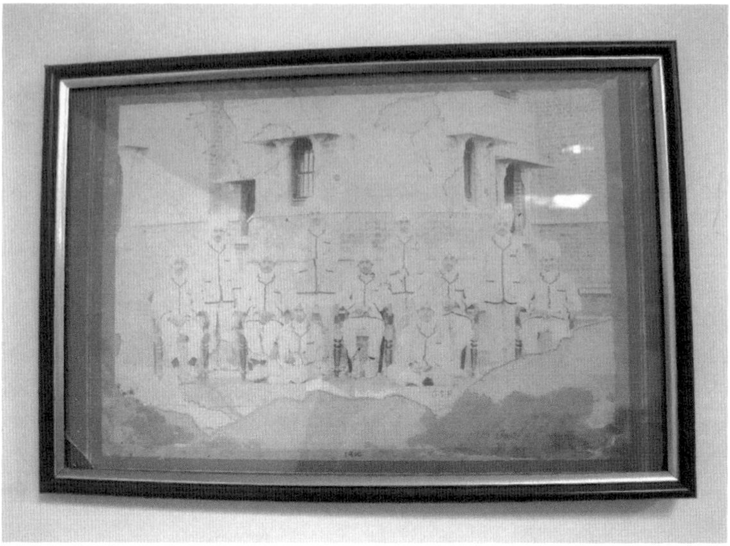

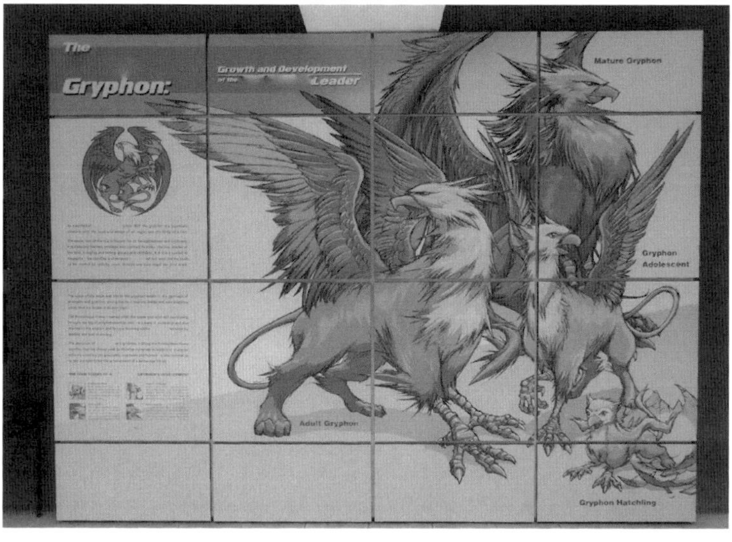
The
Gryphon:
Growth and Development
of the
Leader
Mature Gryphon
Gryphon
Adolescent
Adult Gryphon
Gryphon Hatchling

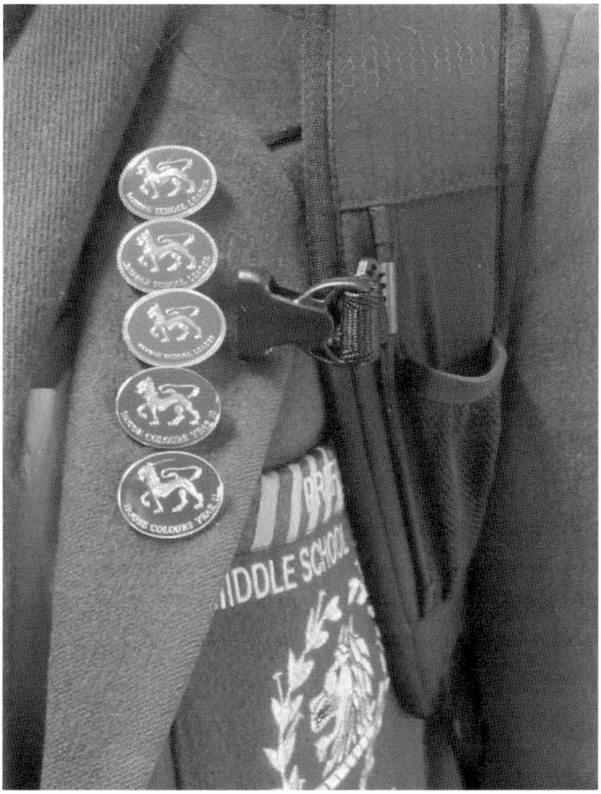

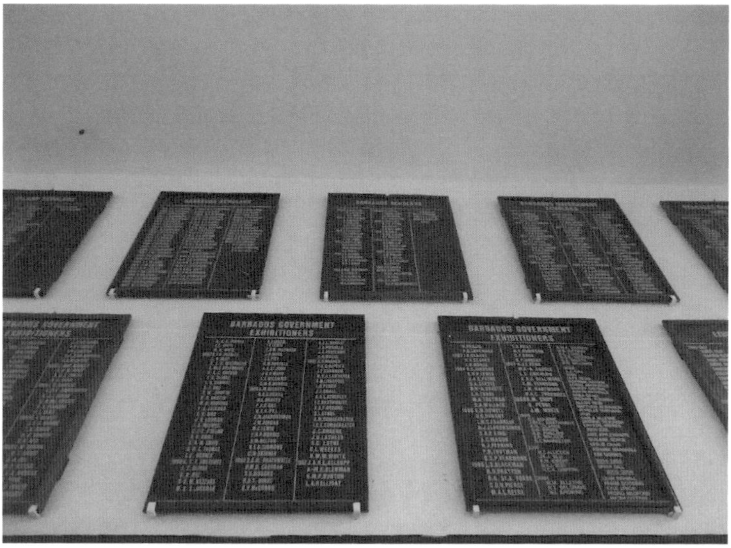
BARBADOS GOVERNMENT
EXHIBITIONERS
BARBADOS GOVERNMENT
EXHIBITIONERS

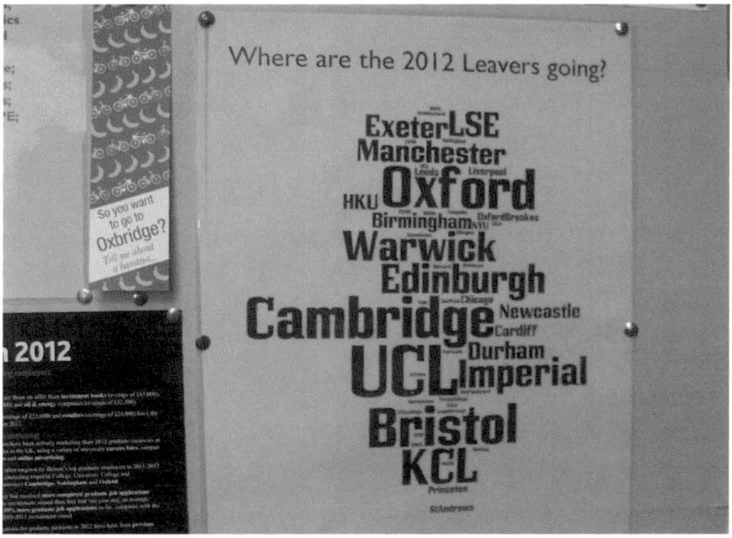
So you want to go to Oxbridge?
2012
Where are the 2012 Leavers going?
Exeter
LSE
Manchester
Leeds
Liverpool
HKU
Oxford
Birmingham
NYU
OxfordBrookes
Warwick
Edinburgh
Chicago
Cambridge
Newcastle
Cardiff
Durham
UCL
Imperial
Bristol
KCL
Princeton
StAndrews

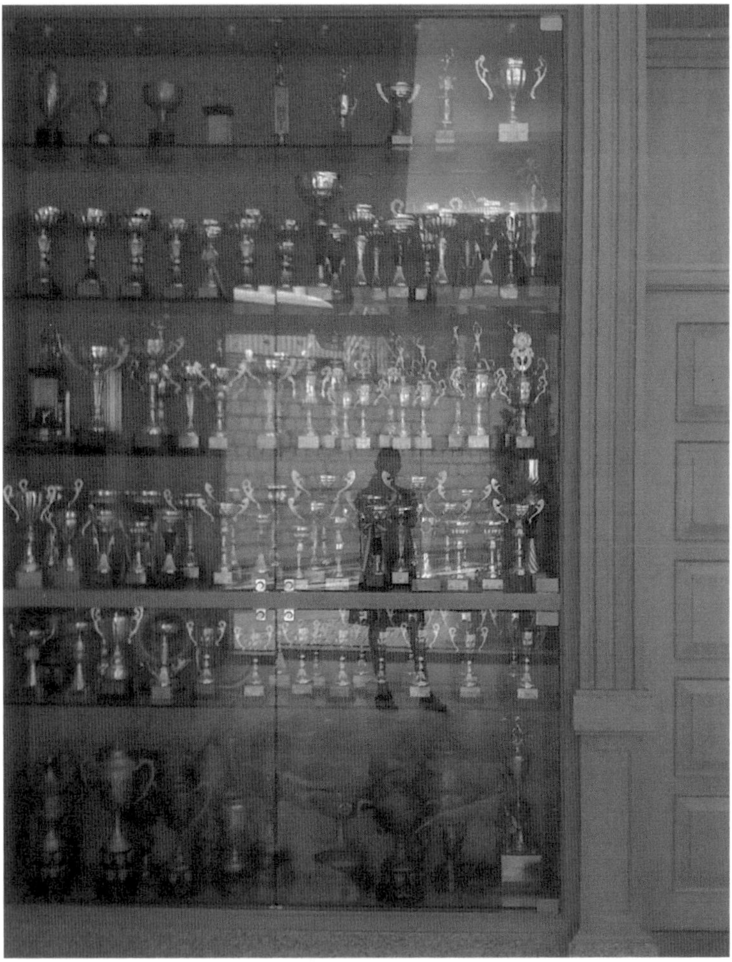

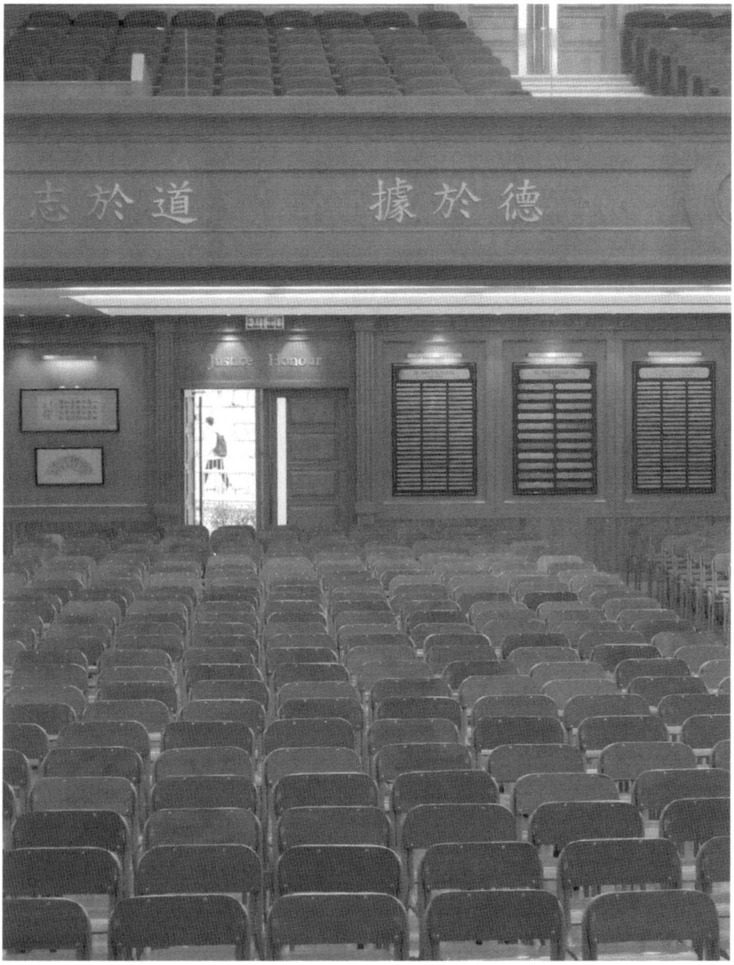

Johannah Fahey is Senior Research Fellow in the Faculty of Education at Monash University, Australia. Her research interests are located in the areas of education and global studies, and are informed by her expertise in cultural studies. She has a national and international reputation in the areas of intersectionality (gender, race and class), and cultural globalization and mobilities. She is the co-editor of Globalizing the Research Imagination (Routledge 2009); and co-author/author of Haunting the Knowledge Economy (Routledge 2006) and David Noonan: Before and Now (Thames & Hudson 2004). She has also published in many eminent international journals and edited books. She is the leading Research Fellow on the international team conducting the research project called Elite independent schools in globalising circumstances: a multi-sited global ethnography.

Vignette: Sound

Johannah Fahey

> Every [student] thinks of the School as he knew it and looks at it through his own eyes. He remembers his own experiences, his own particular friends, the other boys of his time … In other words, he covers the bones of the outlines with the flesh of his own experiences.
>
> Headmaster of Old Cloisters, 1923–1948

The flesh of Sherwood Lashley's experiences as a student at Old Cloisters in the mid-1960s and early 1970s is decidedly monochrome, as it is colored in black and white. He recalls in particular an event that has had a lasting resonance for him. It has remained prominent in the crowd of memories of his school days as it summarily evokes the broader social stratification in Barbados at this time. Having walked to school, Sherwood would stand under the welcome shade of the sandbox tree waiting for assembly to begin. It was here, in the main quadrangle, that he witnessed the same occurrence day after day. Every morning a gleaming Rolls Royce would slowly purr through the school gates and down the tree-lined road, stopping at exactly the point where the doors to the assembly hall opened. At precisely the moment when the bell rang and the school assembly began, the chauffer, who was a black person (like Sherwood) and whom he distinctly remembers wearing white gloves, would open the car door. It was only then that his white student passenger would emerge and immediately make his way up the steps into the cool, quiet recesses of the school hall.

Today many Old Cloisters students (whose population is now predominantly black children) catch public transport to school: there is an array of big blue and gold buses run by the government, but also privately operated minivans. The minivans were my preferred forms of transport while I was on the island and on my regular morning commute to Old Cloisters I noticed that it was generally local Barbadians (including Old Cloisters students), not the heavy traffic of American and

J. Fahey (✉)
Monash University, Melbourne, Australia
e-mail: johannah.fahey@monash.edu

J. Fahey et al. (eds.), *In the Realm of the Senses,* Cultural Studies and Transdisciplinarity in Education, DOI 10.1007/978-981-287-350-7_7

British tourists, who used the minivans to get around. On many occasions I found myself crammed into these vehicles, pressed sweaty shoulder to shoulder with my fellow passengers, or sometimes even sitting on a stranger's knee, the drivers obviously trying to capitalize by accommodating the greatest number of commuters possible. Speeding along at a breakneck pace, the crystal Caribbean sea became a mere blue blur, the sound of the waves crashing upon the shore silenced by the van's incessant horn, clattery exhaust and a booming Ragga soca soundtrack.

One day, when I was walking on a school procession marking Founder's Day with the students and teachers of Old Cloisters we passed through the minivan terminus to get to the nearby church where a commemorative service was being held. The terminus was hot and dusty, a chaotic lot punctuated by the clamorous comings and goings of vehicles servicing different routes around the island. There was a surrounding cluster of tin shacks that sold food and drinks, SIM cards and bootlegged films. There was also an abundance of stray dogs on the street and numerous makeshift market stalls that sold local fruit and vegetables. As I walked with Monica, an English teacher at the school, our conversation turned to van culture, with me exalting the merits of the minivan as a form of transportation. Monica in response said: 'Van culture is representative of all the unsavory parts of Barbadian society that the parents of Old Cloisters students seek to protect their children from'. When I asked her what was unsavory about the minivans, she curtly replied in a statement that terminated our conversation: 'they are loud'.

Reading the social aesthetics of class in this context involves recognizing the ways in which the sensory dynamics of privilege are intertwined with the circulation of particular values and a system of moral evaluation. The parents of Old Cloisters' students, come to define themselves obliquely, not in terms of what they represent, but only in relation to what they don't perceive themselves to represent. Read euphemistically, the so-called 'loudness' of van culture can be interpreted as an assault on refined senses and good taste, with the seemingly 'unsavory' nature of van culture signifying morally unacceptable and offensive behavior. These comments are clearly laden with moral judgments and assumptions about cultural value. Whereby van culture, defined in relation to what it is not becomes a cipher for excess, danger and the so-called working class.

Johannah Fahey is Senior Research Fellow in the Faculty of Education at Monash University, Australia. Her research interests are located in the areas of education and global studies, and are informed by her expertise in cultural studies. She has a national and international reputation in the areas of intersectionality (gender, race and class), and cultural globalization and mobilities. She is the co-editor of *Globalizing the Research Imagination* (Routledge 2009); and co-author/author of *Haunting the Knowledge Economy* (Routledge 2006) and *David Noonan: Before and Now* (Thames & Hudson 2004). She has also published in many eminent international journals and edited books. She is the leading Research Fellow on the international team conducting the research project called *Elite independent schools in globalising circumstances: a multi-sited global ethnography*.

Cultivating Students' Bodies: Producing Physical, Poetic and Sociopolitical Subjectivities in Elite Schools

Johannah Fahey and Matthew Shaw

Introduction

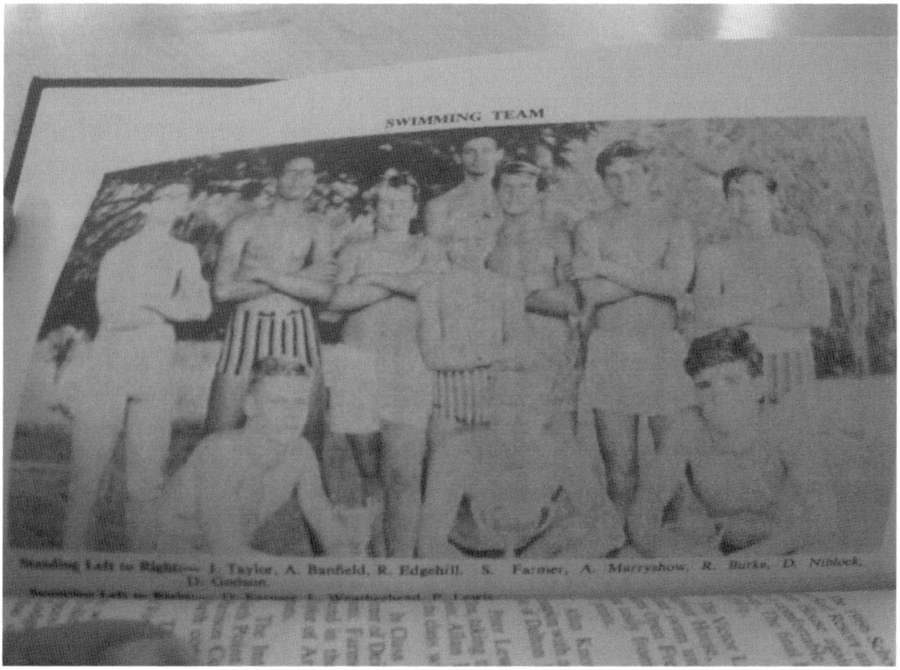

Fig. 1 Old Cloisters' yearbook with a photograph taken in the 1960s of the swimming team

J. Fahey (✉) · M. Shaw
Monash University, Melbourne, Australia
e-mail: johannah.fahey@monash.edu

M. Shaw
e-mail: matthew.shaw@monash.edu

J. Fahey et al. (eds.), *In the Realm of the Senses*, Cultural Studies and Transdisciplinarity in Education, DOI 10.1007/978-981-287-350-7_8

> Aesthetics from this perspective have less to do with artistic expression and the exercise of taste than with the more mundane and pervasive forms of sensory patterning to be found in society, and the ways in which human beings experience and respond to them. (MacDougall 2007, p. 6)

'Everyone has a little bit of black and a little bit of white in them' (Interview 2010), says the current President of the Old Cloisters' Alumni Association. As such, it is problematic to talk about race in terms of black and white in Barbados today.[1] Nevertheless, Jalecia and Rashana, both Old Cloisters' students, talk about the commonplace discussions they have had with their friends regarding living 'a white life' or 'a black life' in Barbados (Interview 2012; Fig. 1). In this respect, embodied identities and the sensory values assigned to them that ascribe certain patterns play an important role in the aesthetics of these girls' everyday lives. Jalecia and Rashana make a distinction based on race between a black life and a white life and a particular form of socializing i.e. social class. Jalecia describes a 'white life' as one involving 'playing polo and tennis, off-roading, swimming and surfing, and going to the yacht club and the races' (Interview 2012; Fig. 1). In contrast to the multifarious activities that a 'white life' affords one, when both girls were asked to describe a 'black life', they said in unison and without hesitation that it involves one thing alone: 'an emphasis on education' (Interview 2012; Fig. 2). Rashana then said 'although we know white students at Old Cloisters, we probably wouldn't see them outside of school because of the different lifestyles they lead' (Interview 2012).

Drawing on cultural anthropologist Arjun Appadurai's (2013, p. 66) suggestion that 'histories produce geographies and not vice versa' (the acknowledgement that geographies are produced over time by 'historical agents, institutions, actors and powers') in this chapter, we will begin by mapping out a wider terrain and examining the histories of British colonialism in the context of Barbados and Cyprus.[2] In this respect, British colonialism can be thought of as having 'circulate[d] through different trajectories, generate[d] diverse interpretations, and yield[ed] different and uneven geographies' (Appadurai 2013, p. 67)—the idea that different histories of British colonialism are manifest differently in different places.

In terms of Barbados, British colonialism is historically linked to merchant capitalism, and 'within this capitalist orbit [Barbados] was developed as a slave-based, export-oriented agricultural colony' (Beckles 2007, p. xiii), whereby up to the 1890s sugar exports in Barbados reached over 90% (Downes 2013). In Cyprus, histories have produced a divided geography and difference is defined in terms of the ethnic community to which a person belongs: with Greek Cypriots and Turkish Cypriots

---

[1] We are aware that a strict delineation between 'black' and 'white' Barbadians is also problematic in terms of our discussion. However, although the category 'colored' (i.e. mixed racial ancestry) is sometimes used, it is more often the case that the literature refers to a 'black middle class' and a 'white elite', even today. We also subscribe to these categorizations throughout, despite their obfuscation of racial nuances. In terms of the student population of Old Cloisters, the Chairman of the school board believes 'now it's about 80% blacks and 20% whites'. (Interview 2011)

[2] Johannah Fahey was part of the research team that undertook the fieldwork in Barbados; Matthew Shaw did so in Cyprus.

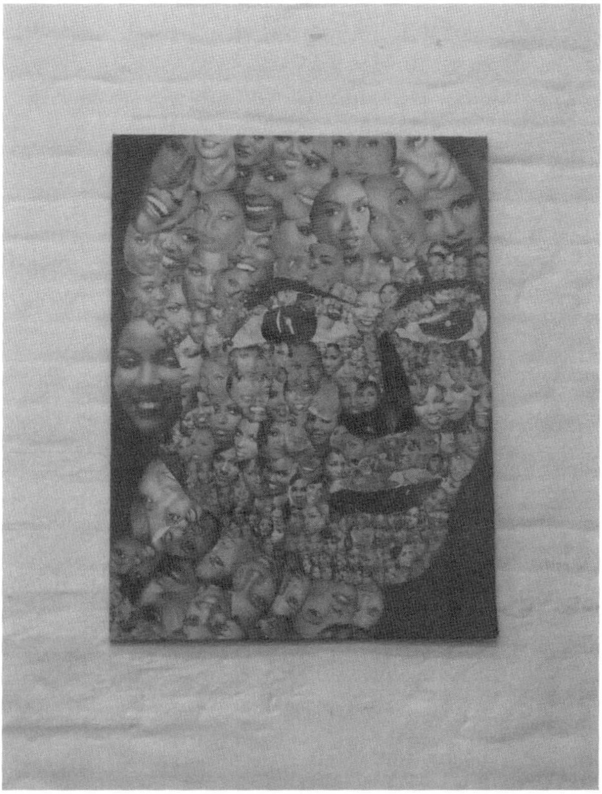

Fig. 2 CXC student artwork

being defined as two distinct communities by the Constitution (Emilianides 2007).[3] History accounts for the boundaries that exist between them, both in the physical landscape of the island and the mental landscapes of the peoples. Recognition of the two communities as being distinct from one another is due to the various different colonialisms the island has experienced during its history which have served to create a highly complicated society, with the island divided on religious, linguistic and ethnic lines. As one student from The Lefkos Academy (TLA; Fig. 3) said, 'I don't know what it means to be Cypriot. I am Turkish Cypriot' (Esin interview 2012).

The school's aim, however, is to create a unified student body rather than exacerbating the differences between students that exist within the island. This is not proving easy and, just as the students in Barbados do not see their white classmates outside of school, nor do the Cypriot students mix in the schoolyard. If you know which students belong to which community, it is noticeable that during breaks there is little interaction between the two bodies of students (Danielle interview 2011).

[3] There are other groups on the island with their own particular identity but they have long made up less than 5 % of the total population so have not been either as politically or socially important as the two largest groups.

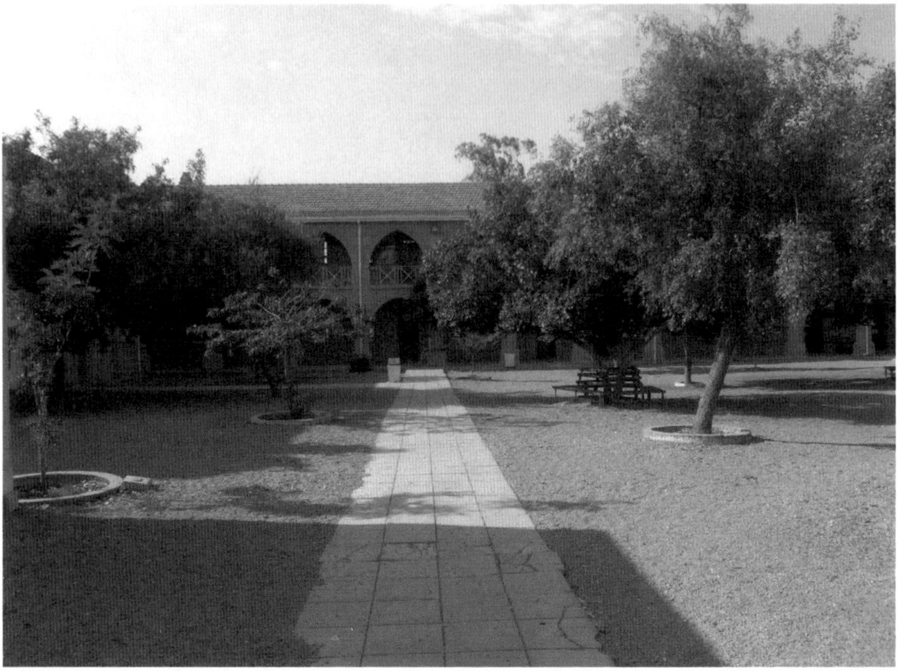

Fig. 3 TLA

When talking about colonial capitalism in South Africa, the cultural theorist Stuart Hall (1980, p. 308) says:

> racial structures cannot be understood adequately outside the framework of quite specific sets of economic relations … one must deal with the historical specificity of race in the modern world. Here one is then obliged to agree that race relations are directly linked with economic processes: historically with the epochs of conquest, colonization and mercantilist domination…the problem here is not whether economic structures are relevant to racial divisions but how the two are theoretically connected.

In terms of colonial capitalism in Barbados and the sensory patterns of Caribbean social stratification, traditional correlations between white skins and privilege and black skins and poverty do not necessarily apply. Rather, as Lamming (2002, p. 85) states, in Barbados social stratification 'is not just between white and black. It is very strong *within*; there is a monolithic white world in Barbados. There was a very strong social stratification *in* that world'. Indeed, during colonial rule in Barbados, 'poor whites [were] thought of as being at the lowest rung of the social ladder' (Lewis 2001, pp. 172–173). In the Cypriot communities racial constructions are not relevant, though the construction of difference based on a person's ethnicity, as marked by linguistic and religious differences, are—since these are what define difference in Cyprus and belonging to one community or the other. Howe (2008) states that colonized cultures were very often resilient and the effects of colonial power patchy and superficial. This is the case with Cyprus where the languages, religions and customs of the communities have been safeguarded—not only during the period since independence from Britain but also during the British colonial period and the Ottoman hegemony that preceded it.

Developing Appadurai's idea, it is our contention that not only do histories produce geographies, there are also certain types of bodily identities that are historically produced in particular places. The social context provided by British colonialism that shapes and continues to shape embodied identities through particular social institutions and their social ideologies (both of which create certain social aesthetic) with a specific focus on two elite schools, one in Barbados called Old Cloisters and the other in Cyprus called The Lefkos Academy are of primary interest. Notions that these classed, raced, and ethnically divided bodies are constituted by history, neither developing in isolation nor as static entities; but rather to be thought of as socially constructed bodies produced aesthetically, relationally and as always in process.

Intertwined Histories of Global Capitalism and British Colonialism in Barbados

The British Empire claimed Barbados as its own in 1627 when a private English merchant company financed settlement with the support of King Charles I.[4] Barbados was the British Empire's first tropical agricultural colony, initially exporting tobacco (for which quick profits were made until an oversupply in European markets caused prices to drop) and cotton and then between 1640–1660 shifting to the production and exportation of sugar (Watson 2013). During this period of settlement, 'descendants of Welsh, Scottish and Irish families, [were] brought to Barbados as servants by the English' (Lewis 2001, p. 173). White indentured servants continued to be transported to Barbados even after this initial period of English settlement. For example, during the Wars of Three Kingdoms (1639–1651) many Scottish and Irish prisoners of war were sold into indentured servitude and from 1653–1658 (the Cromwellian period in England) nearly 7000 Irish were 'barbadosed' to the island (Watson 2013). As a result, Barbados quickly acquired the largest white population of any of the English colonies in the Americas. 'Prior to the Restoration (1660), indentured labor was cheaper than slave labor' (Beckles 2007, p. 28). Indentured servants were therefore the first sugar plantation workers, their white bodies undoubtedly burning under the relentless Barbadian sun. These toiling bodies provided bonded labor. They did not work for wages, but for food, accommodation, clothing and training. Their indenture documents specified the number of years they would need to work for, after which they would be free.

[4] Settlement of Barbados by the indigenous peoples of the Caribbean [the Arawak] (around the fourth to the seventh centuries AD) obviously predates British settlement, as does Spanish and Portuguese settlement from the late sixteenth to the seventeenth centuries. However, as our discussion is concentrated on the history of British colonialism in Barbados We will not address these histories here.

As the sugar industry began to burgeon and the demand for labor increased, so too did the cost of white labor; it was therefore market forces that determined the rise of black slavery in Barbados. Black slaves were imported in large numbers from the Gold Coast region of Africa in particular, especially from what is today the country of Ghana, and from Nigeria. It is estimated that between 1640 and 1807, some 387,000 Africans were shipped to the island against their will (Watson 2013), working under duress on sugar plantations and gaining nothing in return. Moreover, even after slavery was abolished in Barbados in 1834, 'free' men continued to provide free labor, their 'payment' tiny huts provided by the plantation in which they lived, called 'chattel' houses as they were easily moved off the land (that remained the property of the plantation owners) and reassembled elsewhere.

The Aesthetic Space of the School

The legislature in Barbados was elected locally and was responsible for taxation and domestic policy. Therefore, unlike other British West Indian territories it did not benefit from the paternalism of Crown Colony (i.e. British) government, and 'as a result, the Barbadian government and its economy was in the hands of a small, white and wealthy oligarchy—known as the 'plantocracy'—renowned for their racism [and] their reactionary views' (Chamberlain 2006). Although considered their social inferiors there was concern among the white ruling classes about the continuing economic decline of poor white people. As a means to encourage their upward social mobility schools were established specifically for the education of this indigent population (Lewis 2001). Therefore it is possible to suggest that while there was not a class affiliation between poor and rich white people, there was nonetheless a sense of affinity based on a sensory re/cognition of race (i.e. white skin) that elicited concern and afforded poor white people privileges that were otherwise denied to poor black people. The white elites' advocacy for schools for poor white people was influenced by the Church and driven by a moral responsibility for the less favored; only however, if they were white.

Old Cloisters was a charity school founded in the early 1700s by a Bridgetown merchant for 'poor white boys of the parish'. Over time its student population has changed and these evolutions tend to mirror a wider social history of Barbados. In the early 1800s white planters and merchants needed more qualified workers and rather than sending their children to a more expensive school in England they sent them to Old Cloisters. In this period, Old Cloisters shifted from providing an education for *poor* white boys to providing an education for *wealthy* white boys and a curriculum that responded to these changes with the introduction of the Cambridge matriculation exam in 1871.

Black Upward Mobility

At this time, education was also viewed as having a potentially civilizing influence on black people, whose behavior was viewed by the white elite as being willful and dangerous, and following emancipation in 1834 a few gifted poor black male students were able to attend Old Cloisters. During the post-emancipation period, many former black slaves placed more emphasis on upward mobility and education as a means to combat plantation living, and from the 1880s some black men, those skilled in key laboring jobs such as artisans, carpenters, masons and master-tailors but also merchants and politicians, emerged as a nascent black middle class (Downes 2013). In 1904 black Barbadians migrated to work for the US on the construction of the Panama Canal (15,671 black Barbadians left between 1911–1921) and remittances became a source of income on the island, and a means of economic and social mobility (Beckles 2007). 'By 1930 the pattern of land ownership had changed significantly…Panama money, then, had an effect of heightening differences in the material and social standing of black workers' (Beckles 2007, p. 147). Between 1919 and 1937, labor unions, 'landships' (social organizations that mimicked the organization of the British navy and provided social activities for black people working on plantations) and the revivalist-fundamentalist Christian Church (as opposed to the Anglican Church) contributed to a sense of black social cohesion and the development of a black political movement (Beckles 2007). The political mobility of this black population during this time resulted in the 1937 Labour rebellion that ushered in a period of socio-political change culminating in the attainment of independence in 1966.

In terms of how such sociopolitical shifts were reflected in Old Cloisters and the student population, Blackman (2008) talks about the aftermath of the riots of 1937 and Grantley Adams'[5] insight that challenges against the established order and struggles for racial justice and democracy needed to be waged not with violence but rather 'with intellect and sophistication in the constitutional and political arenas'. Clearly, gaining access to the constitutional and political arenas, by middle class black people, required intellectual leadership and thus a certain level of education. According to Blackman (2008)[6]:

> Of the four institutions in that era offering higher education, i.e. Sixth Form level or beyond, three were ruled out: [one] was still an enclave of the Plantocracy; [another] was primarily a theological seminary, and gender discrimination excluded [the other. Old Cloisters] was the only game in town!

Universal free secondary education was introduced in Barbados in the post-colonial 1960s, and Old Cloisters then opened its doors to all eleven-year-old males on the basis of academic merit and without payment of fees. According to Cross, a historian who attended Old Cloisters and who taught at Old Cloisters for 36 years, this meant that 'the son of a top white manager of a plantation could sit in [Old Cloisters] with the black son of a maid and a sugar worker' (Interview 2011). In other words, as students were no longer excluded from Old Cloisters on the basis of either race *or* class, there was an equalization of opportunity at the school. After the sociopolitical upheavals of the 1960s, Old Cloisters then evolved into one of the most prestigious sixth form secondary schools in the Caribbean, its status largely

---

[5] The first Premier of Barbados from 1953–1958.

[6] As these quotes were taken from a speech marking the founding of Old Cloisters, in the interests of protecting the school's anonymity, the reference will not be provided here.

attributed to the fact that since independence five out of its seven Prime Ministers have been alumni of Old Cloisters.[7]

The Colonialisms of Cyprus

Cyprus was different to many other British colonies since it was ostensibly acquired as a result of an agreement whereby the British promised to protect the Ottoman Empire against Russian aggression in Asia in exchange for the island. The underlying reason of self-interest, however, was that they had decided Cyprus would be the key to protecting their interests in western Asia from the Russian advance (Panteli 1984). During the First World War, Cyprus was annexed by the British and in 1925 the island formally became a Crown Colony. It remained so until independence was granted in 1960.[8]

The Orthodox Christian, ethnically Greek, community and Muslim Turkish community already had long histories on the island prior to the arrival of the British. Those of Greek heritage made up the majority of the populace and traced their roots back to the Greek heroic era (Papadakis 2008). The Ottoman Turks conquered the island in 1571. They delegated some authority over the Orthodox community's life to their religious leaders (Dodd 2010) and the church continued to lead the community after the Ottomans ceded control to the British. Therefore, these distinct community bodies lived together on the island and were developing their own social aesthetics around the rituals and symbols associated with the two different languages and their different religions.

Education was an area that was controlled by the respective communities. Initially this was through the Orthodox and Muslim religious leaders. It was, however, something that developed significantly and quickly after the British arrived. Within 5 years of their arrival the number of schools had doubled and by the beginning of the twentieth century this number had nearly doubled again to 322. The majority of these schools continued to be run by the respective communities without any notable interference from the British authorities. The British supported this since they did not want to have to provide the funds to run them (Dodd 2010).

The British did start to take an active interest in education during the 1920s, however, and assumed control over the curriculum in the 1930s (Persianis 2003) because they had become concerned that rising nationalist and anti-British sentiment were being taught in the communities' schools. They thought that if they influenced the running of the schools, and what was taught, a sense of Britishness could develop and there would be stability (Persianis 2003). They were, however,

[7] It became co-educational in the early 1980s and students still gain entry to the school on the results of a competitive examination.

[8] Two small parts of the island have remained in British hands since 1960. These are the two British military bases, Akrotiri and Dhekalia, in which there are approximately 7500 British military personnel and their families.

interfering in matters that the Cypriot communities wanted to keep to themselves and stability did not result.

TLA and British Colonialism

TLA is Cyprus' oldest and most highly regarded private school, having been established in 1900 by an Anglican clergyman who had recently arrived from England, as an undenominational private school for boys serving all communities on the island (School website[9]). It continues to reserve a number of entrance places for students from both the Turkish Cypriot and Greek Cypriot communities (Danielle interview 2011).

The history of TLA in the colonial period divides into two distinct phases. The first phase was from its establishment until 1936 when it was a private school run by the clergyman without any financial assistance from the colonial government (Fig. 4).

When Oldfield retired, the management and control of the school was handed over to the colonial governor, meaning the school was now directly controlled by the British authorities (School website). This occurred after the colonial government had taken control of the education system on the island and was trying to promote the teaching of English—a purpose TLA was able to serve.

Since independence, changes have occurred in the nature of the school including the admission of female students from the early 1960s and the division of the island in 1974. The vast majority of people from the two communities fled from the

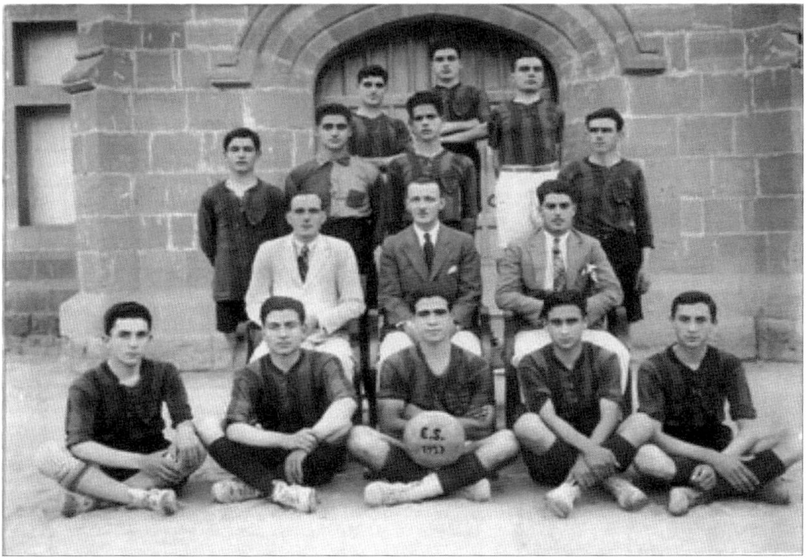

Fig. 4 Photo from the school's earliest days

[9] In the interests of protecting the school's identity, the reference will be anonymized.

other's area of control into that controlled by their own community in 1974, meaning that the places reserved for Turkish Cypriot students were not able to be taken up while the Green Line was closed between 1974 and 2003. In the 29 years they were absent, the school took on a Greek Cypriot character rather than its previous multi-communal one and re-establishing its multi-communal character has proved difficult (Danielle interview 2011). TLA is, therefore, a special case in the Cyprus of today because it is a site where members of both communities share the same space.

From the beginning, entry into the school was selective. The founding clergyman acknowledged that it was difficult to gain a place at the school; partly because 'the payment of fees ke[ept] the school more select' and also because he was 'exceedingly strict in enquiring into the character of boys before admitting them' (Bryant 2004, p. 117 quoting SA1/2766/1904). This meant that students had to display the characteristics that correlated with the British understanding of status, values and behavior. As a result, when he wrote about the dramatic rise in the number of Muslim students, he also stated that he 'refused as many as [he] accepted' (Bryant 2004, p. 117 quoting SA1/2766/1904). This shows that initially the social aesthetics associated with the school were particularly British in character.

This was evident with the introduction of sports such as football and cricket. In these there were expected behavioral characteristics as physical prowess was associated with moral virtue and, although victory was desirable, learning how to cope with setbacks and defeat and not give up was the most important aspect for the development of character (Freeman 2011). Competition prepared students for the battles of life and the moral qualities of respect for others, perseverance, courage, self-control, self-reliance and vigor became an aspect of masculinity and identity in students from these schools that sport was used to develop (Freeman 2011). Participation was meant to be an end in itself and it was the struggle for success which imbued character into the participants. Games, therefore, developed ethical behavior and formed social attitudes that were considered desirable in the group of boys who went to these schools and would then take these attitudes with them into society and, for those that served in colonial administrations, into the colonies. These sports, therefore, created social aesthetics related to the bodies of the students that was British in its nature and applied equally to students from both the Greek Cypriot and Turkish Cypriot communities.

The Geography of Cyprus

TLA is located in the southern part of the island, which is controlled by the Republic of Cyprus, about 3 km south of the Green Line. The Green Line formally divides the Greek Cypriot and Turkish Cypriot communities. Relations between the two communities had been somewhat strained in the decade leading up to independence and this inter-communal unrest turned to violence during the 1960s. Relations between the two communities fractured shortly after independence and, although they did not yet live on a separate half of the island, the Turkish Cypriots had retreated to defined areas in towns and cities after trouble flared in 1963. The complete dislocation of relations occurred in 1974 when the Turkish army landed on the island in response to a coup by a right-wing faction of Greek Cypriots seeking to unify the country with Greece. Many thousands of people were dislocated. Greek Cypriots in the north fled from the advancing Turkish army and Turkish Cypriots in the south also fled or were forcibly sent to the north. As much as one-third of the island's population moved from their homes and there are still many people listed as missing (Athanasopoulos 2001). The island has been divided since that time between the Republic of Cyprus, which is the only official state on the island but only formally controls the approximately two-thirds of the island south of the Green Line, and the area called the Turkish Republic of Northern Cyprus (TRNC) by its inhabitants, which is regarded internationally as a secessionist state only officially recognized by Turkey.

The Green Line is a real, concrete boundary that has reinforced imagined boundaries between the peoples of the communities. As MacDougall notes (2005, p. 127), 'people not only inhabit social spaces but also create them' and, in this case, their creation is both physical and born from the imagination. The boundary was impassible between 1974 and 2003, meaning these social spaces were inhabited in isolation and this created defined sensory worlds for the two groups that were defined by the absence of others as much as those who were present (MacDougall 2005). The dislocation of such a large portion of the island's population continues to define inter-relationships between the communities.

This imagination has been developed by a variety of different social factors, such as schools, families, communities and the media. Kim (Interview 2012), for example, is a Greek Cypriot student whose parents had lived in the north before 1974. She said that she had been at school with Turkish Cypriot students for 5 years before she spoke to one. In her mind, there was nothing to say and the presence of these students meant that more academically worthy Greek Cypriot students who were friends of hers had been unable to get a spot in the school (Kim interview 2012).

The effects of the inter-communal strife after independence and complete disengagement of the two communities after 1974 persist in the imagination of many. The years of separation and the memories of the conflict that led to the division means that stereotypes abound. Students are taught about the troubles in primary school and by their families who lived through them. Esin, when she crosses the Green Line every school day, is entering a society that she did not even know existed until she was 8 years old: 'My mother used to tell me there were people on the other side of the wall but as I had never seen them, I did not believe her' (Interview 2012; Fig. 5).

According to MacDougall (2005, p. 7), the notion of social aesthetics includes 'the geographical setting of a community, and even much in the life of its members that is onerous but to which they become habituated'. It is our contention that histories produce geographies. These geographies then contribute to social aesthetics that functions to construct bodies that are perceived as being different, and therefore separate from one another, on the basis of not just a physical divide, but also a mental division that takes place in the imagination. This creates a sensory experience within the school that affects the social relations between the students and a way of behaving whereby a distance is maintained between many students even though they share a classroom and school yard. These social aesthetics are brought into

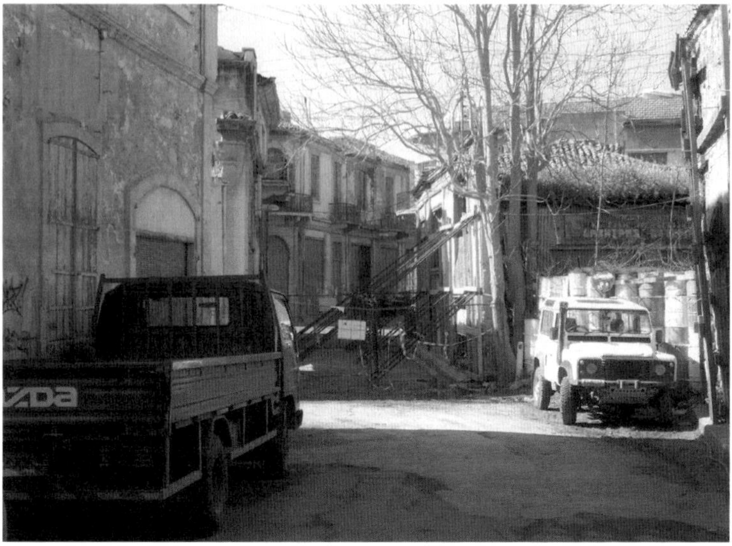

Fig. 5 The Green Line

the school from the community at large and aesthetic patterns are drawn from the identity created by membership of a particular community and how the relationships between the communities have developed in the imaginations of the people in the years of isolation and division. This has created a concrete ethnic divide in the everyday life of Greek Cypriots and Turkish Cypriots. These ethnic origins are decisive as markers of difference between the peoples of the island. These patterns exist within the school, although it is a social aesthetics that the school officially seeks to break down. Sport is one of the conduits through which these official attempts to change social aesthetics are made.

At TLA after independence, students from both communities participated together in school sporting events and Maria stated that within the school when she attended in the late 1960s and early 1970s there was a community feeling and it was not important whether a student was from the Greek Cypriot or Turkish Cypriot community. This was not the case with sport in the wider community at this time. Sport in the wider community was a reflection of relations in the wider community as, by this time, those Turkish Cypriots living in the cities had moved into specific quarters. Then, in 1974, when the division occurred TLA became a Greek Cypriot school in nature as the Turkish Cypriots who lived to the north of the Green Line could not cross into the south. As a result of this separation the social aesthetics of the school took a different form that meant that when the Turkish Cypriot students returned after the Green Line reopened in 2003, they were coming into one that had taken on a Greek Cypriot and Orthodox character with Orthodox religious icons adorning classrooms. Therefore, while the school had maintained its unity before 1974 in spite of the inter-communal tensions in the wider society, the years of isolation and non-contact meant that this has not yet returned in the decade since Turkish

Cypriot students returned to the school. Decisions by the Head Teacher that have allowed Muslim students to observe Muslim holidays have proved controversial and have met with resistance from the school community, especially the Parents' Association (Danielle interview 2011). The prevailing social aesthetic in the Republic of Cyprus seeks to exclude or restrict celebrations at odds with the dominant culture. The school seeks to have an integrated community within its boundaries but the socialization of the students means that this aim is not currently being achieved. The self-imposed exclusion from sport at the school is a way that the Turkish Cypriot students are able to aestheticize their own bodies for use in ways that are meaningful to them but are not consistent with official policy within the school

Old Cloisters Today

> … if the search for identity always involves a search for origins, it is impossible to locate in the Caribbean an origin for its people … questions of identity are always questions about representation. They are always questions about the invention, not simply the discovery, of tradition … The one way in which it is impossible to resolve the problem of identity in the Caribbean is to try to look at it, as if a good look will tell you who the people are. (Hall 2001, pp. 26–27)

As a public school, Old Cloisters is under the Ministry of Education's tutelage and uses the Caribbean Examinations Council (CXC)—a regional examining body that provides examinations for secondary and post-secondary candidates in Caribbean countries—syllabus. The Caribbean Advanced Proficiency Examinations (CAPE) syllabus, which has replaced the Cambridge General Certificate of Education at Advanced Level, is offered largely for students who wish to attend university. Within this program some compulsory subjects have been revised 'to emphasize and state explicitly the link between the syllabus and the creation of the 'Ideal Caribbean Person' (CXC 2010, pp. 39–40; Fig. 6). In brief, the theoretical framework for this policy includes: Wagner's 'survival skills', Gardner's 'multiple intelligence' and Goleman's 'emotional intelligence' (Registrar, Caribbean Examinations Council interview 2011). This policy advocates not simply the production of academic excellence, but egalitarian excellence, a well-rounded or holistic educational excellence embodied in the individual as an ideal Caribbean person.

The Registrar of the CXC talks about his aim to 'Caribbeanize' education (i.e. to offer Caribbean not Cambridge exams) and the role of exams, and the Caribbean 'rethinking its relation to the rest of the world' (Interview 2011). In a recent blog post he says the syllabi is informed by a regional framework 'that forms the basis for a real harmonization of knowledge and standards in the Caribbean' (2012). However, it is worth noting that this harmonization means that both regional universities, and tertiary institutions and external educational institutions in Canada, the United States of America (USA) and United Kingdom (UK) accept the CAPE certification. Obviously, such a qualification has implications for students seeking

Fig. 6 CXC reception

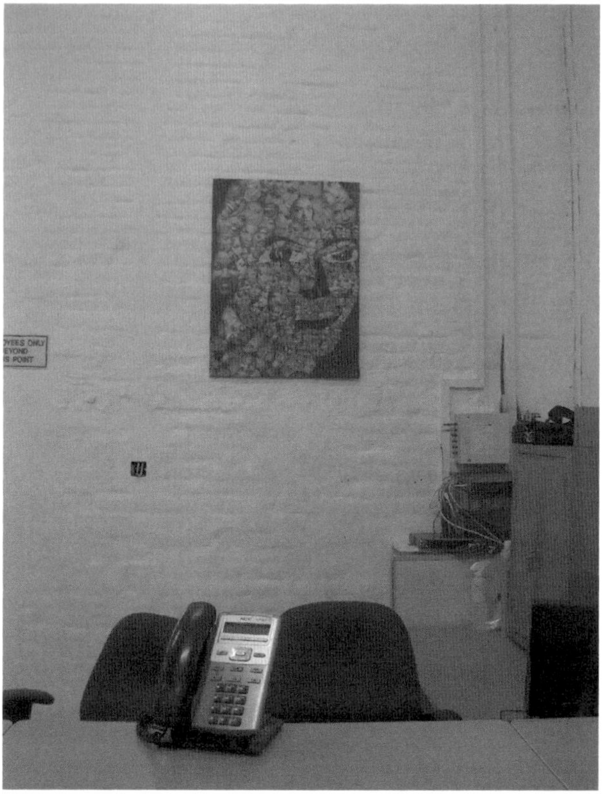

to attend not just regional universities in the Caribbean, but also those abroad, as a means to further their future career opportunities within a global economy.

This emphasis on the region, epitomized by the Caribbeanization of education and the promotion of the ideal Caribbean person has to be viewed through an historical lens. With particular reference to postcolonial Barbados, following independence, the country became 'increasingly immersed within the region's economy and polity, and in fact began to perceive its interests in regional terms' (Beckles 2007, p. 207). In these circumstances, education provided the 'human resources scaffolding that facilitated the modernization thrust' (Jules 2011). More recently, in the past 20 years, the push for the Caribbeanization of education can be seen as a response to what had hitherto been a major driver of educational progress in the Caribbean, that is 'international trends in education that [were] pushed and promulgated by the intellectual financial complex (World Bank, UNESCO, and major donor agencies)' (Jules 2011). As Jules says: 'the essence of the internationalization process is that it leaves little room for small states in particular to fashion an educational paradigm that is significantly divergent from the dominant global one' (2010b).

To see how this policy plays out in practice we now turn to Gabrielle, who is an Old Cloisters student, and how she tactically imagines her embodied identity in the social context of the school's curriculum and the implications of this for her place in a global world. More broadly, the aesthetic dimensions, real or imagined, of body-practices and how this links to the sensory experience of bodies as subjects and the articulation of subjects, the State, history, politics and economy is of interest. Focusing particularly on visual representations of the ideal Caribbean person in the syllabus, and the implications of these representations in the context of the nation, the region and the globe, Gabrielle talks about her art class. (Fig. 7) She says:

> In art the syllabus is designed to control us. And to me art should not be controlled, but they have all these restrictions. The artwork you are producing has to have a Caribbean theme. It has to be a chattel house or palm trees. It is the CXC and on the syllabus it says that you must tie your artwork back to the Caribbean in some way. In my work I did a self-portrait and I just tied a madras scarf around my head and called it 'Creole'. The other thing is that you can do something African and they will consider it Caribbean. But if you did something Asian, say Chinese or Indian that would be a problem, even though our culture is diverse. The Africans came and then in Trinidad the Indians came and the Chinese came, so I don't see why we can't have our artwork influenced by them. But when it is influenced by Africans, it's considered Caribbean too. (Interview 2011)

Fig. 7 CXC student artwork

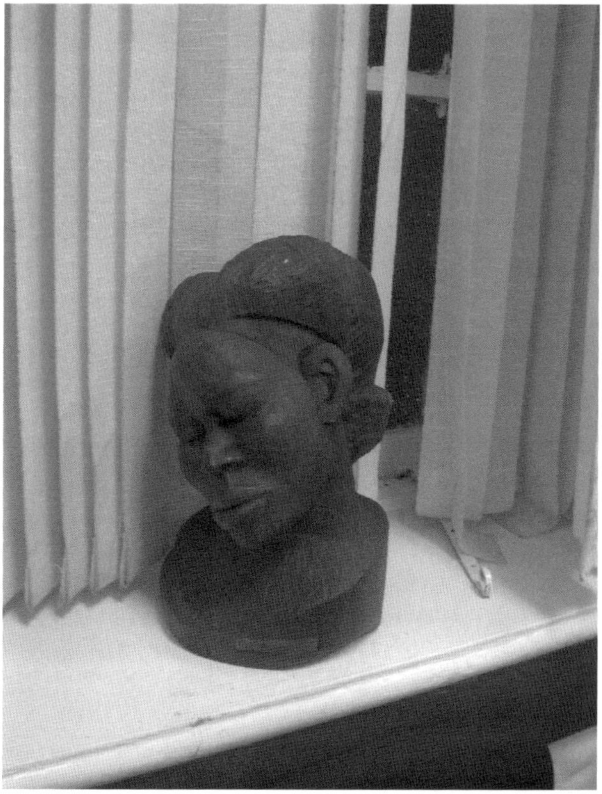

Here Gabrielle draws attention to the tendency within the curriculum to elide the diversity and hybridity of Barbadian identity, not simply into a unified Caribbean identity, but also an integrated African or 'black' identity. This cultural essentialization or racialization of Barbadian bodies is representative of what we would call tactical social aesthetics whereby a subject's embodied identity is linked to a particular aesthetically produced racial identity

Caribbean Consciousness

Hall maintains that 'the question of what constitutes a Caribbean cultural identity has been of extraordinary importance' (1980, p. 26). Talking about the significance of African or 'black' identity with respect to populations that have suffered from the dislocations of conquest, colonization and slavery, he states:

> the first process ... has been the retention of old customs, the retention of cultural traits from Africa; customs and traditions that were retained in and through slavery, in plantation, in religion, partly in language, in folk customs, in music, in dance, in all those forms of expressive culture that allowed men and women to survive the trauma of slavery. (1980, p. 29)

He suggests it is important to associate 'Caribbean consciousness with the African past' (1980, p. 32) as a symbolic means through which black people can 'retell and appropriate their own histories' (1980, p. 26). Speaking of contemporary Barbados more specifically, although a powerful black political elite govern the polity Barbadian whites nonetheless control the Barbadian economy (Beckles 2010). This is despite the fact that only 4% of Barbadians are white (most of whom are descendants of slave owners). C. O. Williams is a key actor in Barbados' white ruling elite. One of the biggest property developers on the island, some of his property includes industrial parks, a recycling center, shopping malls, and a multi-million dollar golf course. He also owns the islands major construction, engineering and excavation companies, and numerous other key industries. It would be erroneous to suggest that C. O. Williams' wealth was inherited from his rich slave owner ancestors, as he is in fact descended from poor white people. However, it is not wrong to suggest that there are sensory histories of white privilege in Barbados, even among the poor. For example, white servants were considered the 'labor elite of the plantation economy' (Beckles 2007, p. 32), and poor white people were the first to benefit from institutionalized education in schools set up between 1733 and 1826 that excluded not only black slaves, but also free black people (Beckles 2007).

Barbados has the dubious history of being a British colony under uninterrupted colonial governance for the longest period of time, from 1627 until 1966. As a country, it was dominated for nearly 400 years by British colonialism and a political and social ideology that depersonalized the majority black ethnic population. As a result, according to Lewis:

> White domination in Barbados has been so deeply ingrained in the socialization process of culture, beginning in slavery and ending in colonialism, that a certain acceptance and internalization of the status quo of the system of race relations is inevitable. (2001, p. 163)

Indeed, this socialization process is in evidence at Old Cloisters today, as Jalecia's and Rashana's comments suggest. When I talked to the President of the Old Cloisters' Alumni Association, who is white, he tended to reiterate the notion that nowadays there was a noticeable delineation in Barbados, based on race and class. This tends to suggest that the 'very strong social stratification between poor and rich whites' alluded to previously by Lamming no longer exists. When we looked at the motto for Old Cloisters together, the President said 'See how island is 'insula', well this island is very insular indeed' (Interview 2010). He then spoke about 'a very strong circle of local white Barbadians, who send their children to private schools [that cater largely to white locals or international students] or to boarding school in Canada' (Interview 2010). He also told me that while he was at a polo match on the weekend he made the observation that almost all of the people there were white.

In Barbados today there is a disparity of wealth between the majority black population and the minority white population. As Cross says, 'the whites still dominate this country in terms of the commanding rights of the economy' (Interview 2012). There is also social stratification between white Barbadians and black Barbadians, as evidenced by the examples given above. Therefore, in this context, the CXC's promotion of the 'ideal Caribbean person' through the valorization of an African connection in its syllabus must be viewed as not just an important economic regionalism strategy, but also an important sociopolitical strategy that takes Barbadian histories into account: the haunting legacies of British colonialism and black slavery and a resulting 'accommodation of white economic power' by black Barbadians over a sustained period of time.

TLA Today

> ...the weight of an institution exists as much in the massed bodies of its members as in the rituals they perform, the traditions they observe, or the material setting they inhabit. A school without its students is a ghost of itself. Moreover, human beings are not merely a physical ballast (although this is important) but a social and psychological presence, the sum of their different backgrounds and personalities. (MacDougall 2006, p. 127)

Ghosts thrive in the Cypriot landscape. There are the ghosts of those missing after the Greek coup and subsequent Turkish 'invasion', or 'intervention'. These people are absent, yet it is an 'absent presence' since the memory of the events that have created the presence remain prominent in the life of the island. The ghost town of Varosha is another absent presence—once the island's holiday center, it is now merely crumbling buildings uninhabited and largely untouched since its populace fled from the Turkish army in 1974. There are the ghosts of those considered martyrs in the struggles of the 1950s when EOKA (Ethniki Organosis Kyprion Agoniston—National Organization of Cypriot Fighters) fought to get the British off the island. Their continued presence is celebrated in statues to the cause, including one particular ghost who was a TLA alumnus. His statue is located meters from the main entrance to the school and is draped in wreathes, with the Greek colors, on the anniversary of his execution.

This statue is a monument to the various identities that the school has and struggles with today. It is a school that seeks to promote unity. Both the Head Teachers to whom I spoke stressed the desire to have the students from the Greek Cypriot and Turkish Cypriot communities view themselves in collegial terms rather than ethnic divisions. Yet the prominent place of the statue at the front of the school, as well as a memorial in the alumni clubhouse, shows that he is an alumnus to be celebrated. His cause, however, was specifically Greek, with his victim being British and the aim of EOKA being to bring the island under Greek rule—another ghost of the island's past (Fig. 8).

The school has been a colonial school, multi-communal school and Greek Cypriot school and these histories converge to create a contemporary community that is finding it difficult to bring together the strands of its history and recreate its multi-communal mandate. It is also unique in that it is a fee paying school that receives funding from the government. Unlike all other schools that receive government funding, however, the medium of instruction is English and it delivers a UK curriculum, the International GCSE, with the aim of having its graduates being accepted into universities outside of Cyprus (School website).

In addition to these ghosts of the past is the ghost of today—the Turkish Republic of Northern Cyprus, which covers one-third of the island and is inhabited by approximately 300,000 people. Yet, as one Turkish Cypriot student at the school,

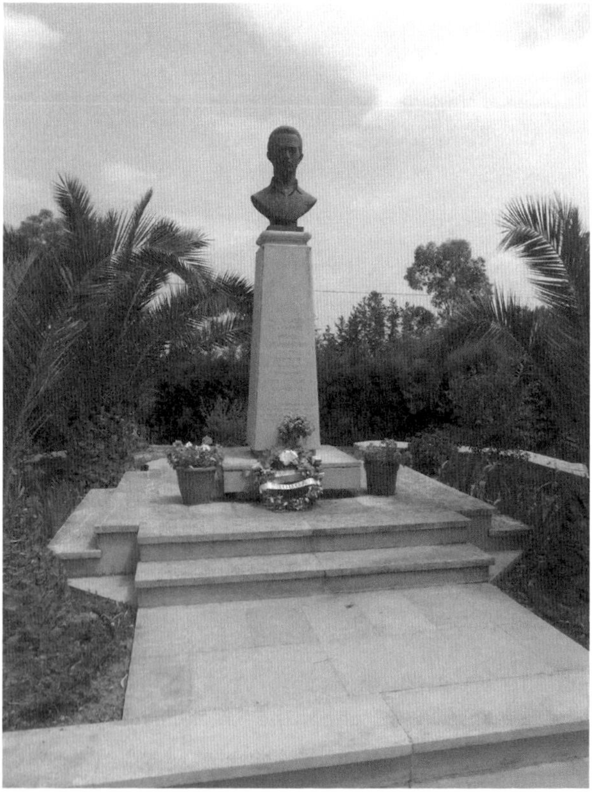

Fig. 8 Statue of executed alumnus

Esin, says, 'I come from a country that does not exist' (Interview 2012). This is an absence from the international community that is a significant presence in the geography of the island itself. Therefore, there is a social aesthetics of absences and 'absent presences' that provides symbolic meaning to the members of the two communities by forming of social spaces that help to define individuals' sense of belonging (MacDougall 2005)

In terms of Esin's identity, she clearly identifies herself as Turkish Cypriot rather than Cypriot (Interview 2012). The two groups live on the island as two peoples. However, upon meeting Greek Cypriots she noticed cultural similarities in the music, food and gestures—more similarities than she noticed with Turks on her travels to Turkey. Nevertheless, it is the differences in language, religion and origin that are emphasized most strongly, reinforcing that there are different social aesthetics at work within each community that maintain the division.

There is a sense amongst Turkish Cypriots that coming from a country that does not exist means they are constantly apologizing for their own existence. In one class discussion about living in Cyprus, one student stated that he thought that, as a community, they allowed themselves to be cast as victims. He perceived this as a weakness that created complexes within the community about how others thought of them and was an impediment to finding a solution to the isolation that those in the north felt as people in an unrecognized state (Hakan interview 2012). To Esin, this sense of not belonging to the globalcommunity in the same way as her Greek Cypriot classmates meant that she saw her future ambitions tied to the resolution of the division of her homeland (Interview 2012).

The social aesthetics of Cypriot society, therefore, are aesthetics of division and absence: an everyday existence where boundaries abound, where borders order notions of belonging, where even the imagination has been largely constrained within these physical boundaries so that the 'Cyprus problem' and the side of the border on which you live defines not only a social environment but also mental parameters.

Sport is meant to be a means of breaking through these mental parameters and promoting unity. When the United Nations declared 2005 as the Year of Sport, Kofi Annan stated that:

> At its best sport can bring people together, no matter what their origin, background, religious beliefs or economic status. And when young people participate in sports or have access to physical education, they can experience real exhilaration even as they learn the ideals of teamwork and tolerance. (Annan 2005)

Although not related, this ties in with other events around this time. In 2004, Turkish Cypriots were again admitted to TLA after the Green Line had been opened by the Turkish Cypriot authorities. The Annan Plan was also put to the populace of the island as a blueprint for reunification in 2004. It was accepted by the majority of voters in the north, but comprehensively defeated in the south since it was believed to be conceding far too much to the secessionist regime (Varnava and Faustmann 2009). Therefore, attempts to bring the Cypriot peoples together were already in vogue by 2005 but meeting with mixed results. The use of sport as a tool for unity can only be meaningful when there is substance to back up the words (Sugden 2010). At TLA, this substance was proving problematic and this reflected the role of sport on the island even in the lead up to independence. For example, when the

Cypriot football league had been established between the world wars, both Greek Cypriot and Turkish Cypriot sides played in it against one another. However, during the EOKA push for independence from Britain and union with Greece in the 1950s, the Turkish Cypriot teams had left and formed a league of their own.[10] Therefore, the separation of identities was evident prior to independence and continued in the early years of independence and sport was a means of consolidating this. The fractured relations between the communities was then most clearly formalized in 1974.

The Turkish Cypriot students to whom I spoke do enjoy sport. Most of them, however, do not enjoy sport at the school and prefer to return to the north to participate in sport. This, therefore, reinforces their own individual sense of their identity within their community, without sport contributing to bringing them together with other students that share their classrooms. Sport, according to MacDougall (2005) is one of the social aesthetic structures within a school that is prominent in student's lives. At TLA, all students are meant to participate in afternoon games (School website) although academic pressures mean that the upper level students are readily exempt (Danielle interview 2011).

The school's inter-house athletics carnival provided a close-up of a wider issue in the school and Cypriot society—the action and inaction of relations between members of the island's two main communities and the nature of their inter-relationships at school, in society and through sport were evident throughout the week-long carnival. The carnival was a demonstration of a ritualized activity from the opening ceremony to the running of the events to the acknowledgement of the individual victors and the champion house. The opening ceremony drew on the Greek origins of the original Olympic Games, representing displays of historical identity and artistic expression. The athletic events represented the purpose of the carnival and provided a display of physical activity while the ceremonies for the victors were a public display. All these activities combined provide socially aesthetic representations of the role of sport as a means of unifying the student body for the single purpose (MacDougall 2005).

However, at the first afternoon of the House athletics carnival the Head Teacher, Mr. Bromhead, asked privately where the Turkish Cypriot students were as all the competitors were Greek Cypriots. Subsequent afternoons were the same. Even though there was meant to be a unifying principle to sport in the school, the self-withdrawal of the Turkish Cypriot students was more in keeping with the isolation and lack of belonging they felt in the southern part of the island in which they were being educated. The participation of athletes from one community and non-participation those from the other reflects the sensory patterns of inclusions and exclusion evident throughout the island.

On the final day all students were present, even those not competing—unlike the afternoon events earlier in the week. Most gathered in small friendship groups and talked amongst themselves. The Turkish Cypriots gathered in one of these groups. It was not totally segregated as they had gathered in amongst other groups of students

[10] There are different perspectives on whether the Turkish Cypriots withdrew or were excluded from the league as both communities have different versions of events. See (Menary 2010, pp. 253–254) and Kartakoullis and Loizou 2009.

and there were civil, casual interactions throughout the day between Greek Cypriots and Turkish Cypriots. However, for the most part they just ignored one another. Therefore, although sport is conducted in the name of 'team ethics' and 'bringing people together', this is proving difficult in practice and division and disinterest, but not disturbance, are the social aesthetics that govern the two communities.

Cypriot Consciousness

At TLA, creating unity amongst its students from all communities is meant to be an antidote to conflict. In Danielle, the former Head Teacher's, words, the school 'is a test case for the unification of the island'. The success or failure of bringing together Greek Cypriot and Turkish Cypriot students is considered to be a guide to how such a bringing together would work in wider society (Danielle interview 2011). Participation in sport is one means of doing this and is also a means of the bringing the physical bodies of the students together to work for a common goal within a sporting environment (Fig. 9). As already mentioned, the UN and sporting bodies, such as the Olympic movement, promote it as a means of allowing peoples from across boundaries to come together. The International Olympic Committee (IOC) (2013), for example, espouses an ideology which aims to 'build a better world through sport' with "sport for all', 'forging friendship amongst athletes' and promoting 'peace through sport' all being Olympic movement ideals (International Olympic Committe (2013).

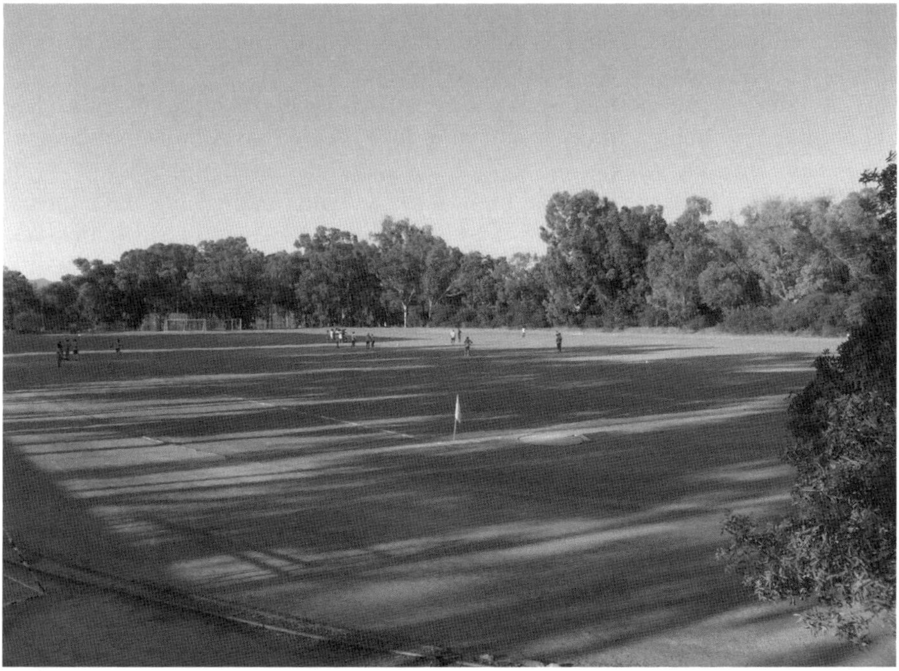

Fig. 9 Sport in action on the school's grounds

These ideals are not, however, only those of a high-profile organization like the IOC. There are many other smaller sporting organizations, such as the PeacePlayers International (PPI), operating in Cyprus since 2006, who also subscribe to them (Tuohey and Cognato 2011). This organization aims to 'unite, educate and inspire young people in divided communities through basketball', which is the specific sport they use (PeacePlayers International 2013). The aim is to involve individuals in their sporting program who might be excluded from other programs (Tuohey and Cognato 2011). This is important for Cyprus because the larger sporting bodies, such as the IOC do not recognize the Turkish Republic of Northern Cyprus and are unlikely to any time in the near future because of political factors.

The PeacePlayers, however, are active on the ground in Cyprus running year-round activities in the hope that having students compete with one another will help to bridge the divides between them and change perceptions that exist within the different Cypriot communities about one another (PeacePlayers International 2013). TLA is one of the sites in which the PeacePlayers operate and students of both ethnicities are members of the same team.

The attempts, however, have not always been successful in practice because, although they can run the program, those within the school or community itself need to support the goals of the program as well. Sport actually fails to break down the boundaries at the school because not all of the staff involved buy into the ethos of inclusiveness. According to the former Head Teacher, Danielle. 'The PE staff are a problem, some of them are very nationalistic and do not want to include the Turkish Cypriot students' (Danielle interview 2011). Conscious efforts are, therefore, being made to create tensions within sport in the school that is contrary to the officially promoted line by the school's leaders. Mr. Bromhead (Interview 2012) spoke enthusiastically about the benefits sport should bring to its participants but then became more careful when discussing its place in the school because of the difficulty in getting all staff to support the school's official sporting ethos.

The attitude of the sport staff was apparent to the Turkish Cypriot students. They did not feel they gained value by attending sports. Esin, for example, said: 'sport is not well run at the school. The staff do not seem interested.' (Interview 2012) A number of other students we spoke to, formally and informally, said similar things. Friendships do, however, develop between students from the two communities. PPI's program specifically seeks to emphasize the 'friendship potential' of its program through repeated, long-term integration (Tuohey and Cognato 2011). However, friendships that do cross these boundaries often prove difficult to maintain because of the social boundaries that persist. According to one teacher at the school:

> The students who make the effort to make friends with Turkish Cypriots find that they lose some of their Greek Cypriot friends as a result. This is because of the extreme nationalist views some students have and vocally proclaim. They, consequently, make it uncomfortable for students who cross the boundaries. (Kevin interview 2012)

The possibility of being ostracized by members of their own ethnic community both within the school and the wider society in which they live means that sport is meeting with limited success in the school in creating enduring relationships.

The solution, therefore, for students who do not feel they are deriving any value from participating in sport at the school—which is the majority of the Turkish Cypriot students—is to withdraw their bodies. This was demonstrated as near enough to all the competitors were at the inter-House athletics carnival were Greek Cypriots. It also emphasized the point made by the Turkish Cypriot students in our class discussion who said they avoided school sport when they could, not because they dislike sport but because of how they feel it is run in the school.

The Cypriot communities, therefore, remain separate and seem destined to develop culturally and economically independently of one another for years to come. They are present together on the island yet a desire to cross the boundaries and form close ties with the other community are largely absent. Whereas Barbados seeks to position itself within its Caribbean region, Cypriots prefer to position themselves within their own community.

Conclusion

Barbados is now a 'service economy' (Downes Interview 2010) spanning tourism, financial and business services, property development, etc. This would explain why C. O. Williams recently built the Port St Charles mariner that includes million dollar apartments offering a 'luxury lifestyle' to tourists. As a service economy, Barbados now needs to focus on the development of human capital. Indeed, human development in Barbados, particularly in the realm of education, cannot be considered without also taking into account economic factors determined by a highly competitive global environment.

In this respect, it is possible to see that the content of the students' artwork at Old Cloisters is intrinsically linked to the curriculum's promotion of an 'ideal Caribbean' identity, as a means for the State to leverage regional affiliation in the students. Presumably this will help to build the country's economic capacity as human capital is harnessed as a resource through a sense of national attachment and thus the flow of students away from the region is stemmed. It is a way for this small island, caught in the 'hurricane of globalization' (Jules 2010a, p. 3), to compete economically on a global scale. As Jules maintains:

> Increasingly notions of national curricula are yielding way to 'foreign' or international curricula that literally prepares a student even from the primary stage 'for export' (packaged as seamless entry) into tertiary education institutions located in OECD centers. This is in direct contradiction to the effort by many nation states to utilize curriculum at primary and secondary levels to help shape nationalist identification and build citizenship. (Jules 2011)

Like many of the students at Old Cloisters nowadays, Gabrielle is not from a wealthy family background. Therefore whilst she would like to study at a university abroad, universities in Canada, the US and the UK are not an option for her because of the costs involved. Gabrielle is aware that she could study at the University of the West Indies, she even suggests that this is implicitly encouraged by the fact that it is very easy to apply, 'you just need to provide transcripts' she says. However, as she dislikes 'the small island mentality' that is characteristic of Barbados, she is still keen to study overseas. One possible opportunity, for Gabrielle, is to study in China, as the Chinese government offers generous scholarships to Barbadian students, which cover tuition, living expenses and even train tickets. If she is accepted into one of the Chinese academies to which she has applied, she will spend the first year learning Chinese in China.

Returning to the Africanization of Gabrielle's artwork, while the historical impetus for CXC's policy promoting the 'ideal Caribbean person' is apparent, particularly in terms of responding to histories of British colonialism and globalization, and while such a strategy is undoubtedly well intentioned, it nonetheless has complex effects on the ground. On the one hand, the Registrar of CXC talks about challenging the 'short-sightedness of our current insularist ambitions' (2013). On the other hand, for Gabrielle, one concern she has, that she thinks will disadvantage her in being accepted into a Chinese university, is about 'the limits of the content of [her] art portfolio'. She says, 'from an outsider's point of view, if you look at my work, it looks like I'm just looking in'(Fig. 10).

Fig. 10 CXC student artwork

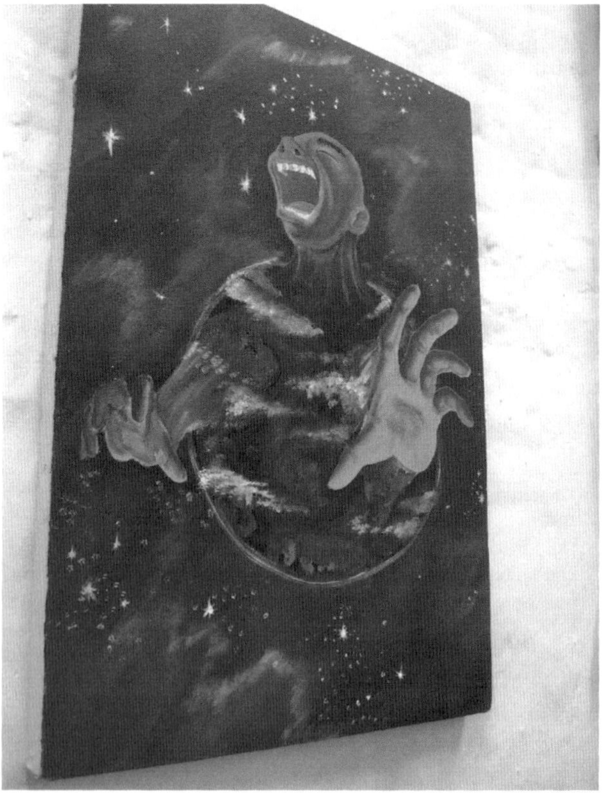

Clearly, the State has to respond to histories of British colonialism and black slavery in Barbados through its policies. However, as Barbados continues to globalize a wider focus on a kaleidoscopic landscape where the State (i.e. Barbados), the region (i.e. the Caribbean) and rest of the world are viewed as having equal socio-political influence, as opposed to a parochial lens trained on its colonial past, needs to be adopted, for as Hall suggests, 'identity is not in the past to be found but in the future to be constructed' (2001, p. 37).

Barbados and Cyprus both wrestle with view focused on the internal. Like Barbados, the Cypriot communities seek to harness the potential of their students. However, the nature of division on the island means that the state remains fixated with a parochial lens, not on its colonial past as such, but on the post-colonial struggle that has led to dislocation and division. Identity is currently very much found in the past and the partitioning of the bodies and minds that has constructed it.

While TLA does provide a forum for students from both sides of the Green Line to come together and some friendships do form, the conclusion to be drawn from observations and interviews at the school indicate that the social aesthetics at play at TLA and Cypriot society, as well as those of absence and presence, are the aesthetics of power. MacDougall (2005) notes that this can rarely be distinguished from other social aesthetics expressions, but the interplay between the school's official desire to create a community of inclusiveness for all of its students and the problems of having all staff buy into it is then played out as a power relationship whereby some staff take exclusionary measures that mean the Turkish Cypriot students do not want to participate. The power these students have is the power of decision over their own bodies and, consequently, do not challenge the measures but withdraw voluntarily.

Sporting bodies that promote the ability of sport as an antidote to conflict neglect the ability of people to use games to exclude and isolate such as is evident at TLA. The sporting social aesthetics at TLA are in conflict just as the island is. The school's leadership are enthusiastic about the potential of sport but dismayed at the reality of it on the ground. The involvement of the school in a successful initiate by PPI demonstrates, however, that in the right forum, with the right support provided, sport can fulfil its unifying function and different social aesthetics are created. However, where unifying principles should be used to bring students together from different communities, exclusion through selection and the preferencing of a language that the majority, but not all, speak leads to the minority questioning its sport's value and pursuing their own sporting interests where they can feel included. Since, however, this takes place away from the school after they have crossed back over the Green Line, the boundary between the students persists.

References

Annan, K. (2005). Press release SG/SM/9579. http://www.un.org/News/Press/docs/2004/sgsm9579.doc.htm. Accessed 30 Dec 2013.
Appadurai, A. (2013). *The future as cultural fact: Essays of the global condition*. London: Verso.
Athanasopoulos, H. (2001). *Greece, Turkey and the Aegean Sea: A case study in international law*. Jefferson: McFarland & Co.
Beckles, H. (2007). *A history of Barbados: From Amerindian settlement to Caribbean single market*. Cambridge: Cambridge University Press.
Beckles, T. (2010). Editorial: Spreading the wealth. http://www.nationnews.com/articles/view/editorial-spreading-the-wealth/. Accessed 13 Sept 2013.
Bryant, R. (2004). *Imagining the modern: The cultures of nationalism in Cyprus*. London: Tauris.
Caribbean Examinations Council. (2010). *Annual report*. St Michael Barbados: Caribbean Examinations Council.
Chamberlain, M. (2006). Memories of race and the formation of nation: Barbados 1937–1967. http://bancroft.berkeley.edu/ROHO/wgmn_papers/mary_chamberlain_paper.pdf. Accessed 13 Sept 2013.
Dodd, C. (2010). *The history and politics of the Cyprus conflict*. Basingstoke: Palgrave Macmillan.
Downes, A. (2013). Sugar was key to middle class structure post-Emancipation. http://www.barbadosadvocate.com/newsitem.asp?more=local & NewsID=29990. Accessed 13 Sept 2013.
Emilianides, A. (2007). Cyprus. In G. Robbers (Ed.), *Encyclopedia of world constitutions* (pp. 240–243). New York: Facts on File.
Freeman, W.H. (2011). *Physical education, exercise and sport science in a changing society*. Sudbury: Jones and Bartlett.
Hall, S. (1980). Race, articulation and societies structured in dominance. In *Sociological theories: Race and colonialism* (pp. 305–345). Paris: UNESO.
Hall, S. (2001). Negotiating Caribbean identities. In B. Meekes & F. Lindahl (Eds.), *New Caribbean thought: A reader* (pp. 24–39). Jamaica: University of West Indies Press.
Howe, S. (2008). Empire and ideology. In S. Stockwell (Ed.), *The British empire: Themes and perspectives* (pp. 157–176). Oxford: Blackwell Publishing.
International Olympic Committee. (2013). Olympism in action. http://www.olympic.org/olympism-in-action. Accessed 20 March 2013.
Jules, D. (2010a). School: The last frontier of Caribbean civilization, Old Cloisters Speech Day, Dec.
Jules, D. (2010b). Rethinking education in the Caribbean, Dec 13. http://www.cxc.org/media-centre/registrars_blog. Accessed 12 July 2012.
Jules, D. (2011). Reinventing education in the Caribbean- Part 1, *The Gleaner*, January 26. http://jamaica-gleaner.com/gleaner/20110126/news/news1.html. Accessed on 12 July 2012.
Jules, D. (2012). What does CXC really mean? January 17. http://www.cxc.org/media-centre/registrars_blog. Accessed 12 July 2012.
Jules, D. (2013). The challenges that we face. http://www.cxc.org/?q=node/7595. Accessed 13 Sept 2013.
Kartakoullis, N. L., & Loizou, C. (2009). Is sport (Football) a unifying force or a vehicle to further separation? The case of Cyprus. *The International Journal of the History of Sport, 26*(11), 1652–1667.
Lamming, G. (2002). *The sovereignty of the imagination: An interview with George Lamming*. Durham: Duke University Press.
Lewis, L. (2001). The contestation of race in Barbadian society. In B. Meekes & F. Lindahl (Eds.), *New Caribbean thought: A reader* (pp. 144–195). Jamaica: University of West Indies Press.
MacDougall, D. (2005). Social aesthetics and the Doon School. www.roninfilms.com.au/get/files/955.pd. Accessed 30 Dec 2013.
MacDougall, D. (2006). *The corporeal image: Film, ethnography and the senses*. Princeton: Princeton University Press.
MacDougall, D. (2007). The experience of colour. *The Senses and Society, 2*(1), 5–26.

Menary, S. (2010). Football and the Cyprus conflict. *Soccer and Society, 11*(3), 253–260.
Panteli, S. (1984). A new history of Cyprus: From the earliest times to the present day. London: East-West Publications.
Papadakis, Y. (2008). History education in divided Cyprus: A comparison of Greek Cypriot and Turkish Cypriot schoolbooks on the 'History of Cyprus'. Oslo: International Peace Research Institute.
PeacePlayers International. (2013). Mission, vision and values. http://www.peaceplayersintl.org/about. Accessed 20 March 2012.
Persianis, P. (2003). British colonial higher education policy-making in the 1930s: The case of a plan to establish a university in Cyprus. *Compare, 33,* 351–368.
Sugden, J. (2010). Critical left-realism and sport interventions in divided societies. *International Review for the Sociology of Sport, 45,* 258–272.
Tuohey, B., & Cognato, B. (2011). PeacePlayers international: A case study on the use of sport as a tool for conflict transformation. *SAIS International Review, 31*(1), 51–63.
Varnava, A., & Faustmann, H. (Eds.). (2009). *Reunifying Cyprus: The Annan Plan and beyond.* London: IB Taurus.
Watson, K. (2013). Slavery and economy in Barbados. http://www.bbc.co.uk/history/british/empire_seapower/barbados_01.shtml. Accessed 13 Sept 2013.

Interview Data

Old Cloisters. (2010). President, Old Cloisters' Alumni Association, Barbados.
Cross. (2011). Former Student, Old Cloisters, Barbados.
Gabrielle. (2011). Student, Old Cloisters, Barbados.
Jalecia. (2012). Student, Old Cloisters, Barbados.
Rashana. (2012). Student, Old Cloisters, Barbados.

Barbados

Downes, A. (2010). Professor, University of the West Indies, Barbados.
Downes, A. (2011). Registrar, Caribbean Examinations Council, Barbados.

The Lefkos Academy

Danielle. (2011). Former Head Teacher, The Lefkos Academy, Cyprus.
Esin. (2012). Student, The Lefkos Academy, Cyprus.
Hakan. (2012). Student, The Lefkos Academy, Cyprus.
Kevin. (2012). Teacher, The Lefkos Academy, Cyprus.
Kim. (2012). Student, The Lefkos Academy, Cyprus.

Primary Sources (these have been anonymised)

Blackman, C. (2008) 'XXXX', Lecture delivered on the 275th Anniversary of the Founding of Old Cloisters, April 30. 'XXXX': a second century of excellence. http://www.XXXX.ac.cy/. Accessed 30 June 2014 (The Lefkos Academy website).

Johannah Fahey is Senior Research Fellow in the Faculty of Education at Monash University, Australia. Her research interests are located in the areas of education and global studies, and are informed by her expertise in cultural studies. She has a national and international reputation in the areas of intersectionality (gender, race and class), and cultural globalization and mobilities. She is the co-editor of *Globalizing the Research Imagination* (Routledge 2009); and co-author/author of *Haunting the Knowledge Economy* (Routledge 2006) and *David Noonan: Before and Now* (Thames & Hudson 2004). She has also published in many eminent international journals and edited books. She is the leading Research Fellow on the international team conducting the research project called *Elite independent schools in globalising circumstances: a multi-sited global ethnography.*

Matthew Shaw is a PhD candidate in the Education Faculty at Monash University, Melbourne. His interests lie in history including the history of sport as well as the place of sport in schools and society. His dissertation looks at the role sport has in a divided society and the way it is used to reinforce or break down boundaries.

Visual Essay: Bodies

Johannah Fahey

Affinities and Otherness

Those that underpin the functioning of elite schools deliberately absence themselves, they occupy instead an inconspicuous shadowy realm. This is not an immaterial place as it is fully substantiated by labor: by black workers at Greystone in South Africa who can only bear witness to a passing parade of largely white coiffured girls; by the uniformed staff at Ripon College who are on hand, alert and attentive yet never front and center; by Filipina domestic workers, who are substitute mothers for some of the boys at Cathedral College, and whose rare days off consist of sharing cardboard shelters offering flimsy privacy in the bustling heart of Hong Kong; by staff at the Caledonian School who traverse the liminal space of a car park using a bicycle as a means of transportation; and by a lone worker in an empty classroom at Highbury Hall who is captured as a mere blur in the photographic frame. Within/across elite schools there are similarities and affinities. But there are also differences and otherness constructed according to the class/race/gender triumvirate. Not so much diametrically opposed categories, not simply a matter of black and white (although sometimes this is the case), but rather a mutual reinforcement; based not necessarily on a convenient blindness, but on a distinction between those who command the dominion of sight and those who necessarily remain unseen—the hidden labor that makes privilege possible and the world of the elite school work.

J. Fahey (✉)
Monash University, Melbourne, Australia
e-mail: johannah.fahey@monash.edu

J. Fahey et al. (eds.), *In the Realm of the Senses,* Cultural Studies and Transdisciplinarity in Education, DOI 10.1007/978-981-287-350-7_9

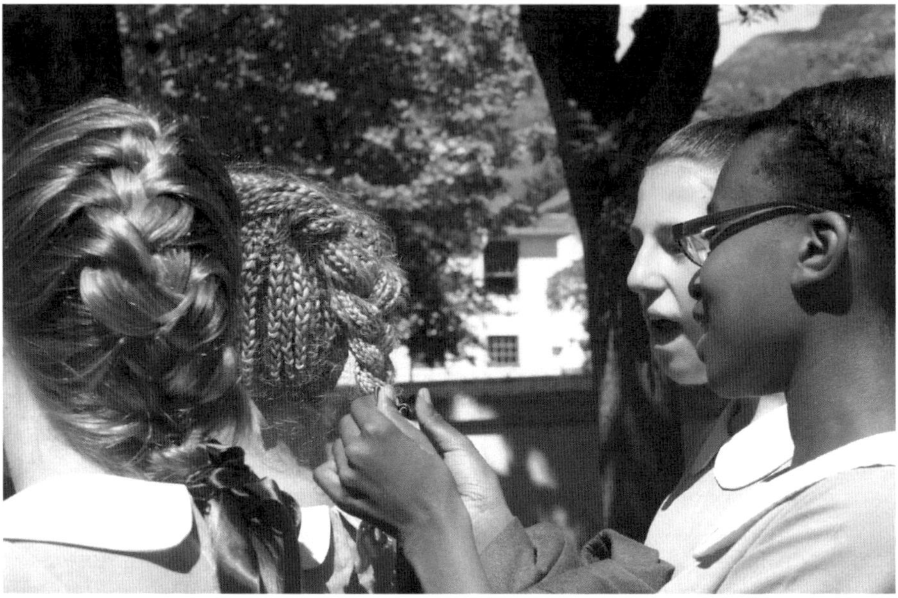

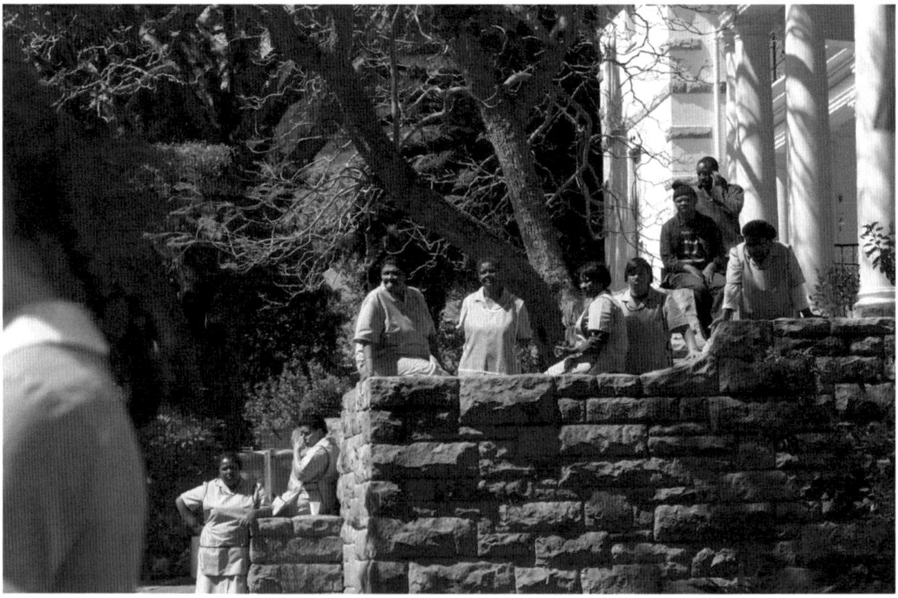

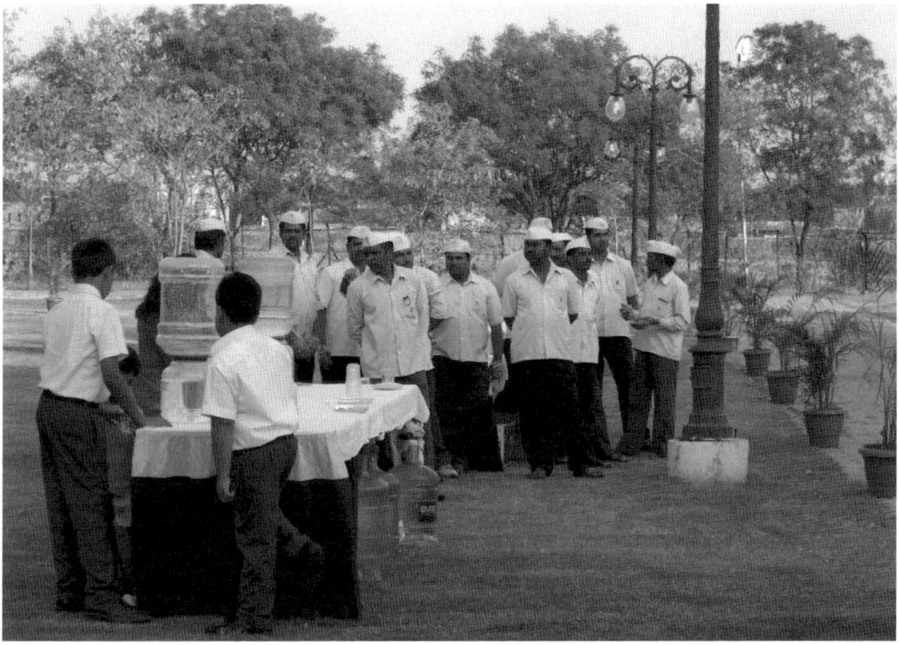

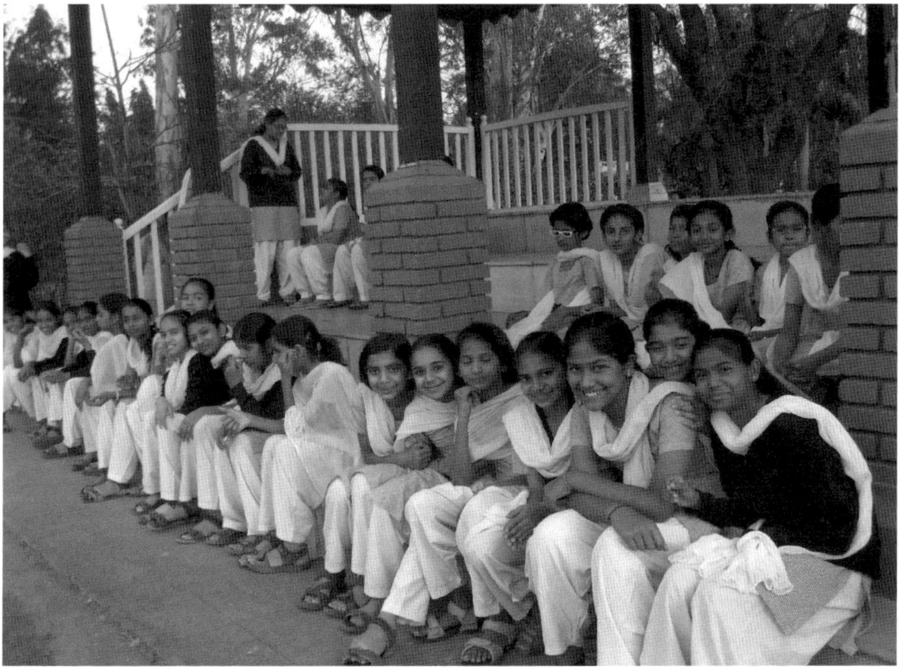

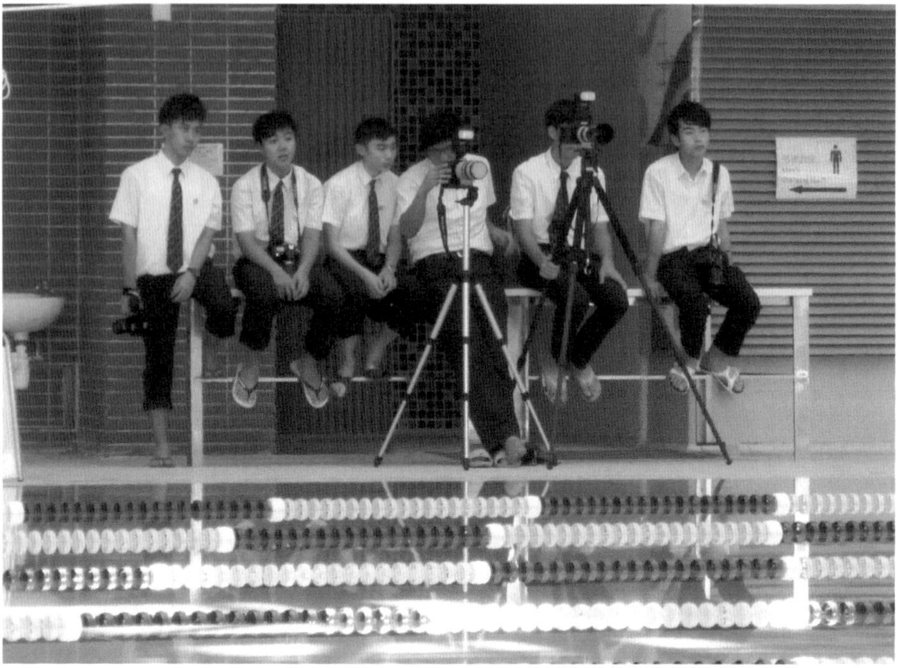

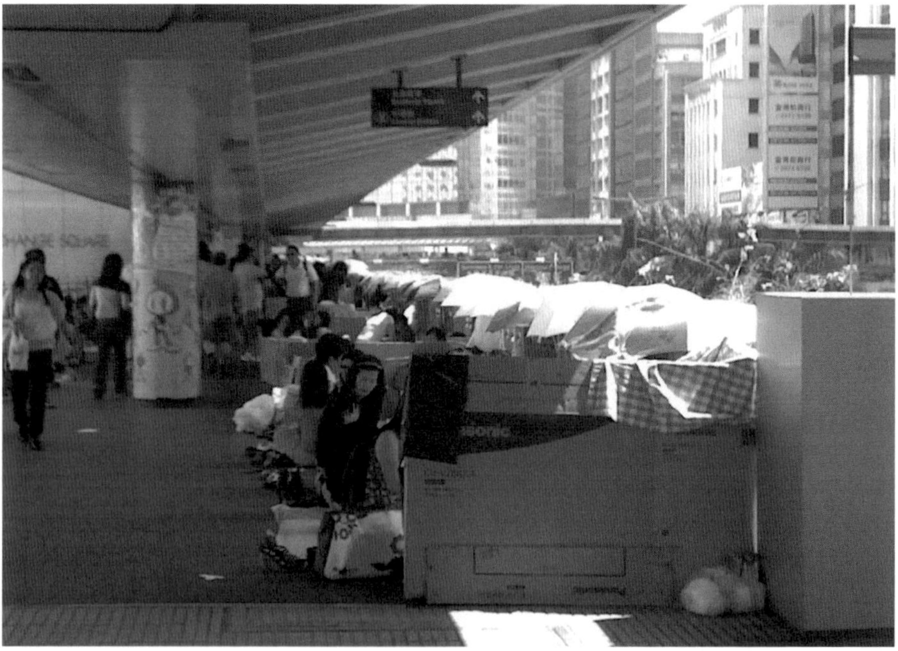

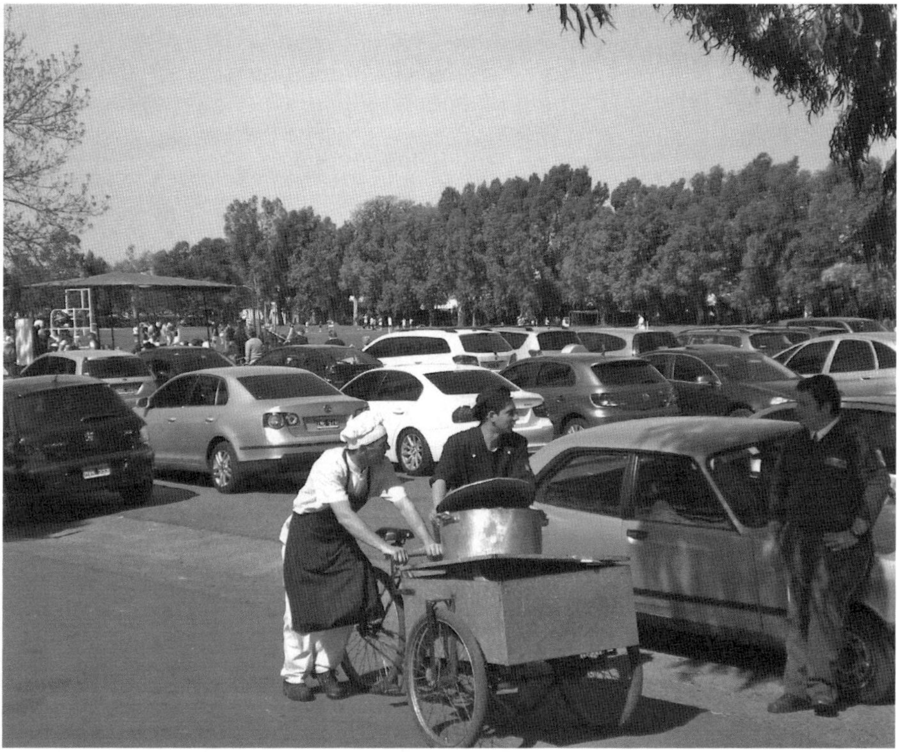

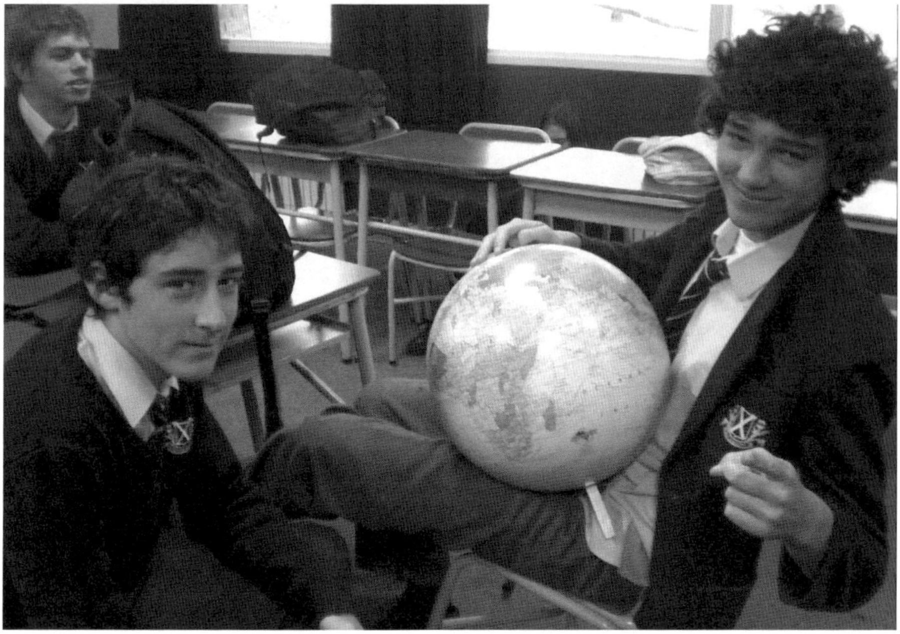

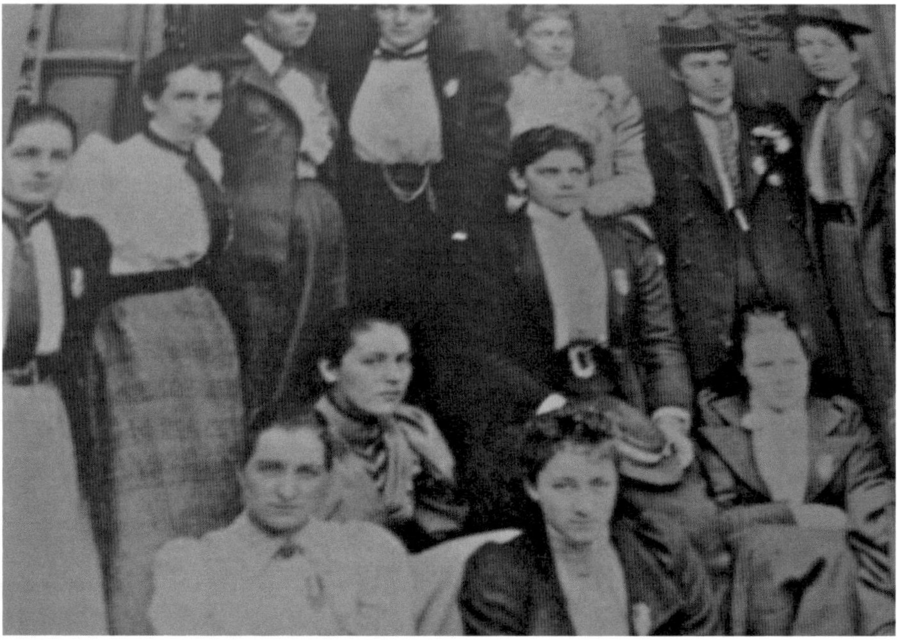

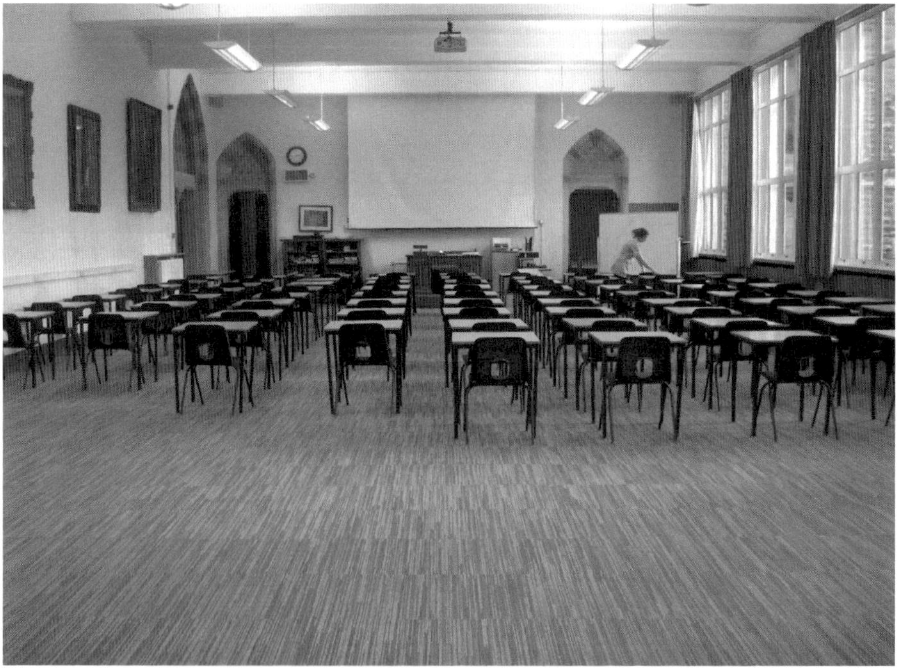

Johannah Fahey is Senior Research Fellow in the Faculty of Education at Monash University, Australia. Her research interests are located in the areas of education and global studies, and are informed by her expertise in cultural studies. She has a national and international reputation in the areas of intersectionality (gender, race and class), and cultural globalization and mobilities. She is the co-editor of Globalizing the Research Imagination (Routledge 2009); and co-author/author of Haunting the Knowledge Economy (Routledge 2006) and David Noonan: Before and Now (Thames and Hudson 2004). She has also published in many eminent international journals and edited books. She is the leading Research Fellow on the international team conducting the research project called Elite independent schools in globalising circumstances: a multi-sited global ethnography.

The Visual Field of Barbadian Elite Schooling: Towards Postcolonial Social Aesthetics

Cameron McCarthy, Heather Greenhalgh-Spencer, Koeli Goel, Chunfeng Lin, Michelle Castro, Brenda Sanya and Ergin Bulut

> What threatens the authority of colonial command is the ambivalence of its address… (Bhaba 1994b, p. 97)
> But a storm is blowing from paradise… (Benjamin 1968, p. 257)

In this chapter, we seek to explore schooling in the postcolonial context as a particular type of cultural artifact (Appadurai 2013). By this, we mean that schools in the so-called developing world are often laden with the markers of the colonial past etched into their material and imaginative practices and resources that situate them in the present and orient them to the future. We explore these 'etchings' by drawing attention to the visual domain of social interaction and cultural production. The visual domain often exists as a postcolonial sublime, under-examined and largely ignored in educational or sociological analysis to date, drawing on MacDougall (2006), we suggest postcolonial social aesthetics (PSA) expose the robust histories captured within the visual. Such is the case with the school whose visual domain is the subject of this chapter—Old Cloisters in Barbados. Eschewing the dominant qualita-

C. McCarthy (✉) · H. Greenhalgh-Spencer · K. Goel · C. Lin · M. Castro · B. Sanya · E. Bulut
University of Illinois at Urbana Champaign, Champaign, USA
e-mail: cmccart1@illinois.edu

H. Greenhalgh-Spencer
Texas Tech University, Lubbock, TX, USA
e-mail: heather.greenhalgh-spencer@ttu.edu

K. Goel
e-mail: koelig21@gmail.com

C. Lin
e-mail: clin59@illinois.edu

M. Castro
e-mail: mccastr2@illinois.edu

B. Sanya
e-mail: sanya2@illinois.edu

E. Bulut
e-mail: erginb@illinois.edu

J. Fahey et al. (eds.), *In the Realm of the Senses,* Cultural Studies and Transdisciplinarity in Education, DOI 10.1007/978-981-287-350-7_10

tive research tendencies (even in the case of critical and radical scholarship such as postcolonial studies) to privilege the word, we examine Old Cloisters as a visual text.

The Word Versus the Expanded Text of the Visual: PSA

Much of postmodern criticism focuses on the word (Derrida 1978). Language and communication are defined as practices that happen through text and talking. Postcolonial studies, even postcolonial ethnographic research, seem similarly transfixed by the word. Ethnographers interview real actors dwelling in the zone of exception of the ethnographically bounded landscape; the research field with its global forces and connections and imaginations are distilled down to what is said, what is told, what is narrated. The ethnographer is like the old colonial police officer of George Orwell's (2014) famous essay *Shooting an Elephant*, a man or woman with a pen and a notebook, all eyes, but especially ears, tuned to the scene of the ethnographic subject. On the cover page of *The Predicament of Culture*, James Clifford (1988), visually presents the ethnographer's dilemma through a photographic enactment of the skit, Onyeocha, ('white man') of Igbo; performed as part of festivals in South East Nigeria. The 'white man' of these performances is an embalmed recorder who euthanizes the world of the native in the text.

We wish to push against the temptation to valorize the word at the expense of the visual. At a time when the anti-aesthetic trend is still prevailing in postcolonial studies, we argue that postcoloniality can be interpreted visually by focusing on a series of photographs of Old Cloisters in Barbados. Specifically, by calling attention to visuality in the postcolonial setting, we are pointing beyond the mere physiological practices of vision toward what we coin here *postcolonial social aesthetics* (PSA). Amalgamating postcoloniality with visuality, PSA connotes critical reflection on the postcolonial society via visuality. More importantly, perhaps, the term denotes the culturally constructed nature of the postcolonial space and the production of differences in relation to human social interactions within the visual furniture and symbolic order of that particular space. That is to say, rather than pointing to vision and the visual as the mere act of seeing, we situate the visual as part of the production of identity and culture in postcolonial spaces. As argued by Henri Lefebvre (1992) in *The Production of Space*, identity and place, and moments in time are made up of complex interactions between ideology, social practice, histories, and materialities. Lefebvre points us to the force of *things*, the force of interactions in place. In order to get at these complex interactions the visual field and an understanding of the social aesthetics at work are necessary. As cultures, arts and societies are increasingly interwoven in an era of globalization, PSA can offer us illuminating insight as to how postcoloniality presents itself, communicates with the people and is understood by means of seeing and representing.

The haunting aspects of the postcolonial past are especially vital for understanding culture and subjectivities. It is through the lingering of the colonial past in the 'postcolonial' moment that we can grasp the rhythms and particularities of the postcolonial space in its dynamic and also almost frozen way that still keeps inspiring the contemporary moment of the school body with its past and ambitions into the future. As MacDougall's (2006, p. 96) work mentions with reference to an ex-student from an elite Indian school, these institutions are such that wherever the students go, they 'will always carry the school' and the colonial and postcolonial past. That is why postcolonial social aesthetics and photography are useful for documenting the moments of performance, play (along), and escape.

Students use their Blackberry digital devices, and other forms and affordances for virtual production and consumption, as a means of escape from the haunting and disciplining past and rhythms of the school. They also show great insight, connection, and experimentation as they 'play' with identity making through both consumption and production of the visual field. This is how, we believe, one can explore the contradictions within the neatly designed 'habitus'[1] of the school setting (Bourdieu 1993). The visual allows us to more fully interact with the nuanced moments and interactions—the ecology—of postcolonial life in the site of the school. Examination of the visual domain weakens the walls of containment Old Cloisters uses to regulate the sacred inside of the school from the profane world outside its perimeters; it allows for a more nuanced and complex understanding of students' lives both inside and outside of the school.

Theoretical Foundations of PSA

Our PSA paradigm owes much to the work of four social and critical theorists, namely, John Berger (*Ways of Seeing*), Walter Benjamin (*The Work of Art in the Age of Its Technological Reproducibility, and Other Writings on Media*), Pierre Bourdieu (*The Field of Cultural Production*), and Homi Bhabha (*The Location of Culture*).

First, the backbone claim of PSA is that seeing is social. In *Ways of Seeing*, Berger (1972) states that:

> The relation between what we see and what we know is never settled. Each evening we *see* the sun set. We *know* that the earth is turning away from it. Yet the knowledge, the explanation, never quite fits the sight [emphasis in the original]. (Berger 1972, p. 7)

Berger (1972) argues that the way we see things is not merely a personal experience, but a social reconstruction process, which is affected by our knowledge and belief. Put another way, seeing is social because 'we never look at just one thing; we are always looking at the relation between things and ourselves,' (Berger 1972, p. 9) and because what we chose to look at or not look at is a social choice. Recognizing that 'seeing comes before words' (Berger 1972, p. 7), Berger emphasizes the role of the visual and seeing in revealing social interactions bewildered in text. Based on

[1] By, habitus we are referring to the sum total of dispositions, values, and meaning of style that are anchored in the deportment, body hexis and everyday practices that define individuals and their relationship to stratified social power and material resources. According to Pierre Bourdieu, habitus is composed of: [s]ystems of durable, transposable dispositions, structured structures predisposed to function as structuring structures, that is, as principles which generate and organize practices and representations that can be objectively adapted to their outcomes without presupposing a conscious aiming at ends or an express mastery of the operations necessary in order to attain them (Bourdieu 1993, p. 5).

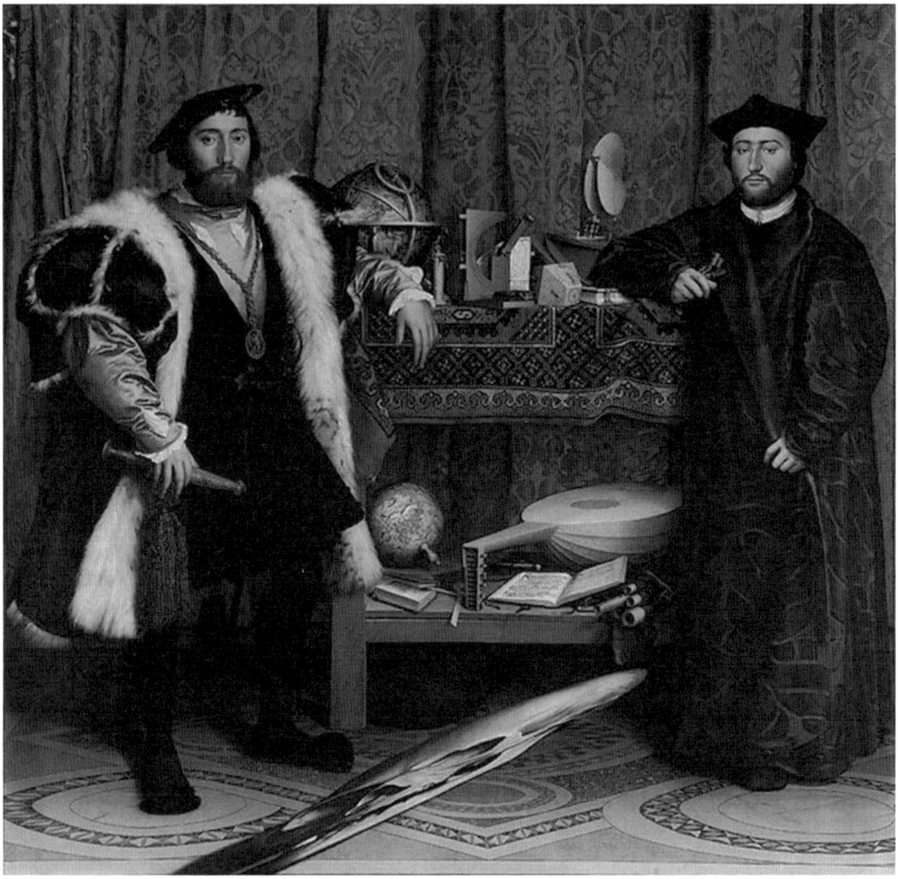

Fig. 1 *The Ambassadors*, Holbein (1533). (This work has been identified as being free of known restrictions under copyright law, including all related and neighboring rights)

the visuality of Hans Holbein's painting, *The Ambassadors* (1533), Berger's (1972) aesthetic analysis of the painting helps interpret the social relation between the colonial conqueror and the colonized (Fig. 1).

In addition to seeing, the sociality within the visual field is also determined by the process of representation, which David Levi Strauss (2003) calls 'aestheticization'. For Levi Strauss (2003, p. 9), 'to represent is to aestheticize'. In other words, aestheticization is a converting process through which imaginings are socially and culturally encoded in order to make them visually and conceptually appealing to others, and thus to make a point.

Second, PSA is built on Walter Benjamin's groundbreaking work on social aesthetics. Benjamin's (2008) social aesthetics approach to analyzing photography is articulated in his essay 'Little History of Photography' in which he advocates to focus not only on the aesthetic value of the photographic work, but also on 'its embeddedness within economic, social, technological, and political practices' (Benjamin 2008, p. 264). Benjamin (2008) develops two concepts, the 'optical unconscious' and the 'aura' as cornerstones of his framework. The optical unconscious refers to the capacity of the photographic image that makes the image-world present itself in a different way from what we see with the naked eye (Benjamin 2008). The aura is regarded as a medium, a determinant and a 'historical variable' (Benjamin 2008, p. 265) in interpreting the image. The aura converges two things: 'the historical conditions of possibility' of the image and a 'self-consciousness of a certain class... at a particular moment of its development' (Benjamin 2008, p. 265). While interpretation of the photographic image is subjective, Benjamin (2008) does recognize what he calls 'image imperatives,' something he considers 'the lessons inherent in the authenticity of the photography' (Benjamin 2008, p. 293), indicating that some information culled from the 'image-world' is objective.

Third, our PSA also borrows ideas from Pierre Bourdieu's theory on the role of culture in the reproduction of social structures and the social uses of photography in particular. Refuting the Kantian notion of the universality of the aesthetic, Bourdieu (1993) introduces the concept of habitus, a notion of the agent. He grounds the agent's action in objective social relations. In other words, to understand the practices of artists, we need to understand two histories first: 'the history of the positions they occupy and the history of their dispositions' (Bourdieu 1993, p. 61), all of which eerily remind us of Benjamin's concept of the aura. For Bourdieu (1993), the perception of artwork jointly involves conscious and unconscious deciphering operations though which concealed power tends to be 'broadly accepted, and often unquestioned' (Bourdieu 1993, p. 2). In addition, Bourdieu (1993) views the artistic field as a field of position-takings and the aesthetic disposition is socially designated, produced, and must be reproduced.

Finally, our PSA is informed by Homi Bhabha's postcolonial theory about the cultural hybridity, translation and re-inscription of modernity on its social imaginary. In *The Location of Culture*, Bhabha (1994, p. 6) notes that: 'postcoloniality, for its part, is a salutary *reminder* of the persistent neo-colonial relations with the 'new' world order and the multinational division of labor'. For us, such a reminder can simply be the visual one. By displaying these photos and putting those visual reminders together we attempt to create what Bhabha (1994, p. 26) terms as 'the temporality of negotiation,' revealing 'the historical connectedness between the subject and object of critique' by means of negotiation through visual messages. Specifically, against the backdrop of postcoloniality, we want to question the fixed frame and the space of representation, to showcase the invisibilities, to bring a range of contradictory, but coexisting places to attention and to re-examine the transnational and translational hybrid location of cultural value by visual methodology under the paradigm of PSA.

The Research Context and Methodology

As noted above, the school that provokes our visual analysis is Old Cloisters, located on the island of Barbados—a fundamentally transnational island. Old Cloisters was established by a planter and merchant in 1733 and from the eighteenth century until the last quarter of the twentieth, it operated as a virtual extension and transplant of the British public school system to the island, which resulted in it being labeled the 'Eton of the West Indies.' For instance all of Old Cloisters' headmasters came from Oxford, Cambridge or London up until 2003, when the current headmaster began his tenure. With all of its headmasters being educated outside of the West Indies for 270 years, Old Cloisters negotiated colonial cultural trappings and postcolonial realities. There are also broad political connections with the school—in that all of Barbados' prime ministers and governor-generals, except two, have been graduates of Old Cloisters. Cutting from the past to the present, the school is now confronted with the new powerful realities of globalization, nationalist and regionalist orientation of the state, its legal incorporation under the ministry of education, and the powerful trumping global imaginations of youngsters who unlike their school's teachers dwell more securely on the internet, feast more fully on electronic relays from the US and negotiate—with perhaps overly-optimistic expectations—the international recruitment offensive of universities from North America into the Barbadian school setting.

With this in mind, we are attending not only to the content of the images—signs and codes—but also the broader social relationships, articulations, global and local connections, and spatial organizations of objects within the image. In this respect, our method is one that is inspired by semiology, as well.

We include photographs culled from several different research trips to this elite school over the course of 2011 and 2012. These photos were taken during our fieldwork in Barbados as part of a larger global ethnography project on global elite schooling. Each photograph we present has become part of our argument about postcoloniality; that meanings can exist apart from or in addition to the original independent meaning of the subjects in the photos. In other words, we foreground the social interaction 'behind the scenes', and beyond the subjects using a PSA perspective. For example, the reason that we include the photos of the Barbados College Fair in our selection is not so much because it records a social event as the fact that it embodies a postcolonial modernity by unfolding a recruitment of Barbadian elite students by North American tertiary education institutions, and what is more, by capturing the interaction between the indecisive young Argonauts and the determined recruiters, we also call attention to the performance and 'playing along' that exists in postcolonial spaces. Likewise, the photo of the scenically stunning beach is selected not to show the natural marvel of the Caribbean Sea; rather, it is intended to zoom in on postcoloniality through a lens of global capitalism. Specifically, what the photo highlights is not a beach in its natural condition, but a globalized postcolonial space that is visually outlined by the stark contrast between the tourist plantation hotel in the background and its consumers—symbolic owners laying under the beach umbrellas—in the foreground, and the 'neo-colonial relation,' in Bhabha's words, between the multinational consumers and what they are consuming.

However, we are not suggesting that a single image can tell everything about postcoloniality. We are not suggesting that all photos must be read in the same way, by everyone. On the contrary, we argue that the reading of these photos is a complex and on-going negotiation process and any fettered 'authentic' interpretations always ought to be avoided. Instead of looking for markers of authenticity, PSA calls for the viewer to notice what is there and what may not be there. PSA attends to the histories and dispositions that help to produce the moment and reveal historical markers shown in the photograph.

Postcoloniality as Visually Encoded Lived Experiences

We argue that the elite school in the postcolonial setting is a site of curation and consecration in which colonial condensations abound along with markers of indigenizing and globalizing registers of change and transformation. These markers are inlaid in the rich imagery of everyday rituals of school life, the artifacts and emblems of school identity, the architectural forms of school buildings, the curricular texts and materials used in the classroom, and the vigorously imaginative universes of real and vicarious action verbalized by students in their interviews with researchers. Yet this is a vibrantly hybrid and contradictory context. We illustrate these hybridities and complexities in the examples of photographs drawn from our visits to Old Cloisters with minimal commentary.

This chapter, both visual essay and textual analysis, seeks to sketch the post situ of the global ethnographic field in a single island or site through recovery of the visual domain of Old Cloisters and its extension into the built landscape. It foregrounds the image and iconography of the postcolonial elite school context stretching it out beyond the school to the ends of the island, the horizon cast by the sea ('the sea ain't got no backdoor' is a Bajan saying of the gentrified working class). A density of hybridities appear in the visual domain, the scenario of the encounter between the colonizer and the colonized gathered in an anthropology of images—a recorded inventory in which history and present, nation and global, native and subject collide in found objects and in the expressive landscape (Williams' *Night and the Olmec* [1983], Harris's *Companions of the Day and* Night [1975]) Each photo is a vignette, a sketch of contradictions, desires and ambitions, riddles of the past dwelling in the built environment, promises of the future fraught with obscurity and absent of guarantees. This attention to the visual field of schooling takes on a particularly heightened significance in the postcolonial school setting, where Old Cloisters literally wrestles with the future in vocabularies of tradition as it seeks to better prepare their students for the transforming circumstances of tertiary education and the transforming occupational choices generated in the global context.

In what follows, we call attention to these stories by showing a paradox of the colonial past in the present and at the perimeter and edge of the island, reading the establishment and the popular from the Fiskean beach inward to the old plantation houses and new tourist plantation hotels as interchangeable and hybrid territory linked to the school itself and its consecration (the school and the plantation house are interchangeable, the school built on the plantation, fossilized in a living inventory, markers of an unrecorded public memory) to its codification of excellence, the summary of its essence in achievement, its cabalism of symbolism and ritual, its metaphors.

The Context: Postcolonial State for Travelers and Tourists

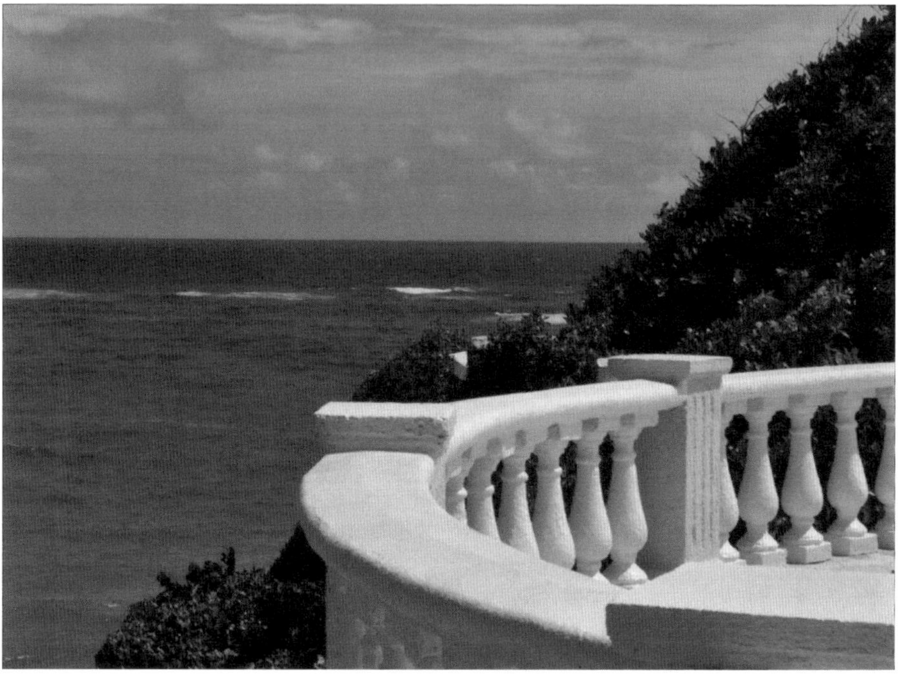

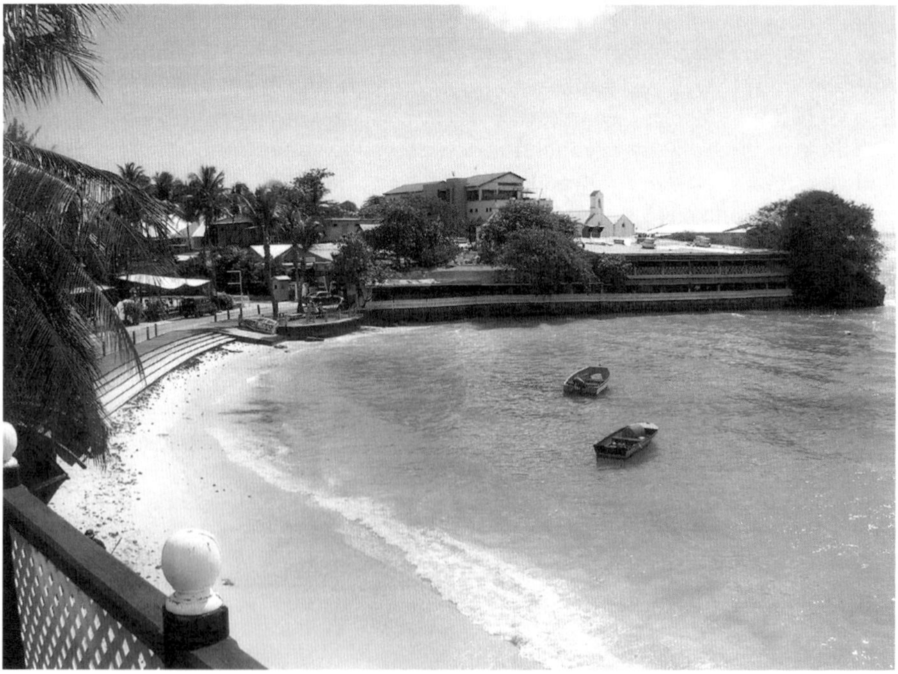

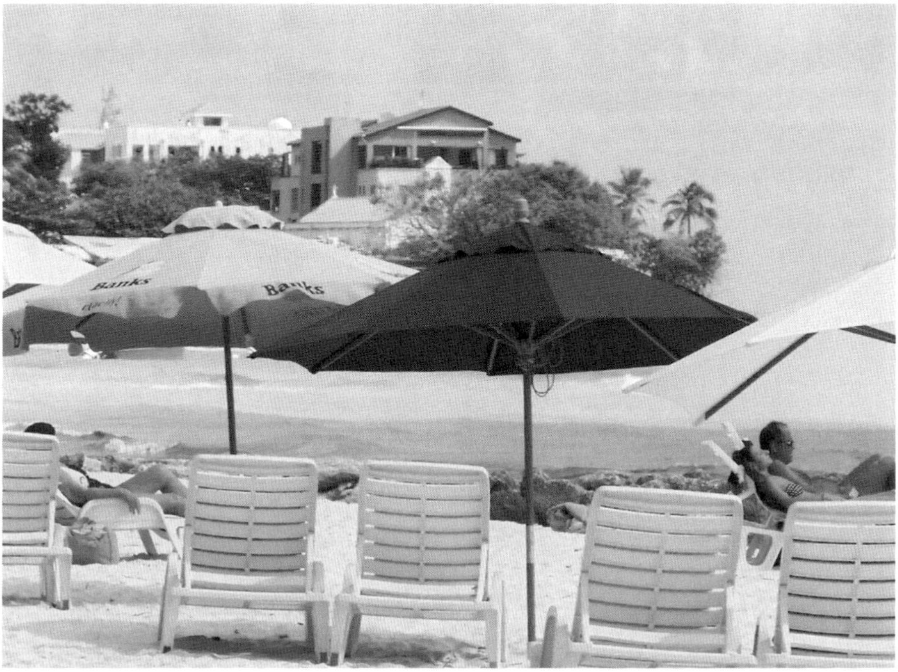
Banks
Banks

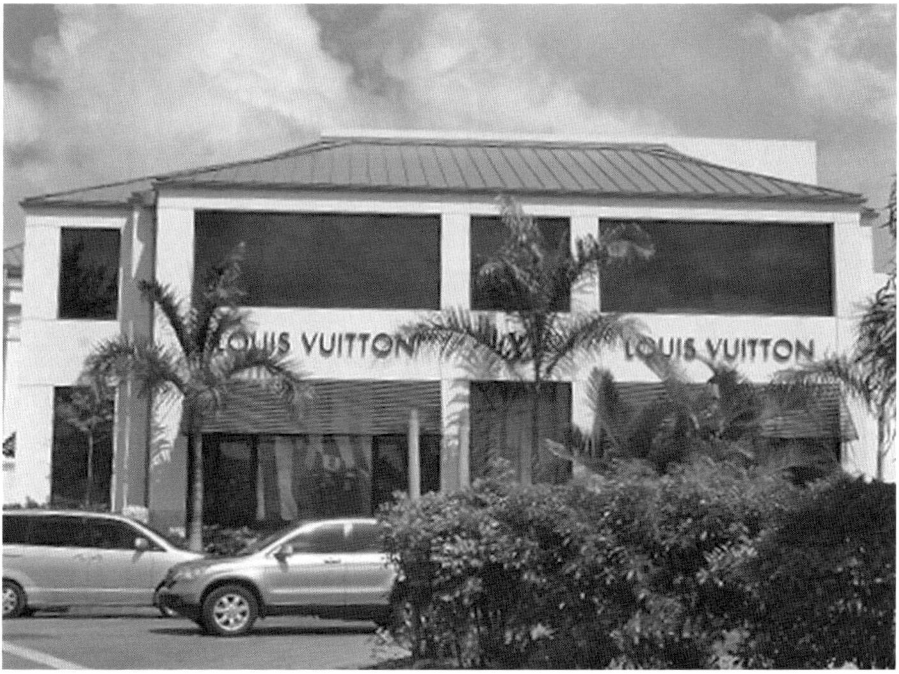
LOUIS VUITTON
LOUIS VUITTON

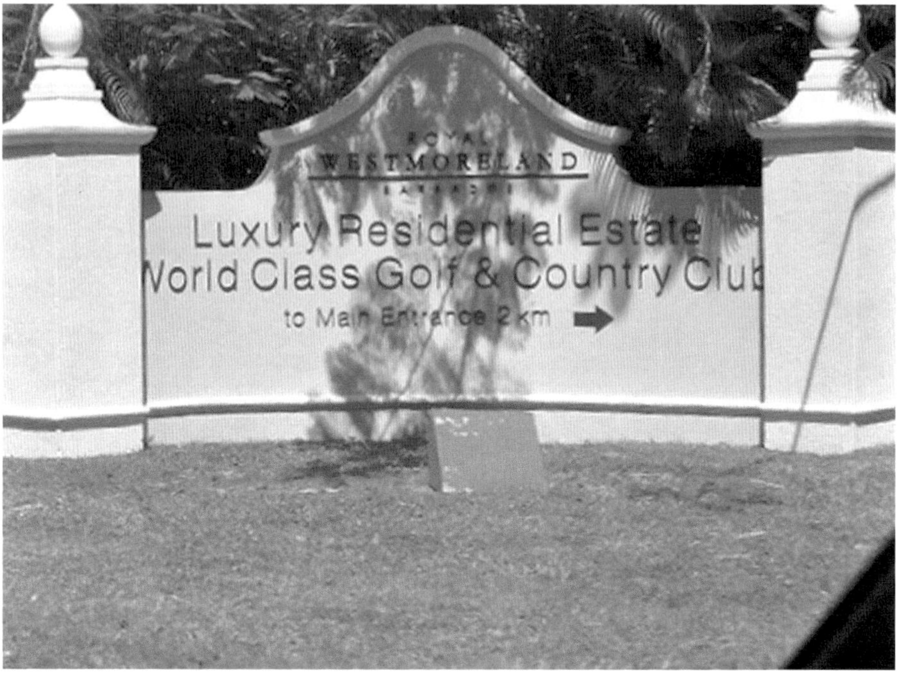
WESTMORELAND
Luxury Residential Estate
orld Class Golf & Country Clu
to Main Entrance 2 km

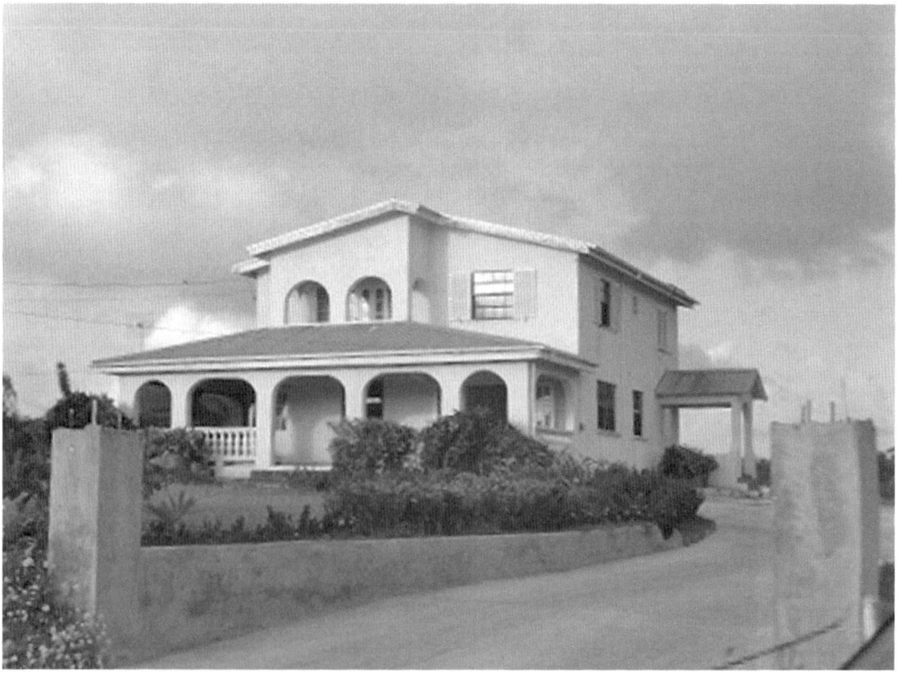

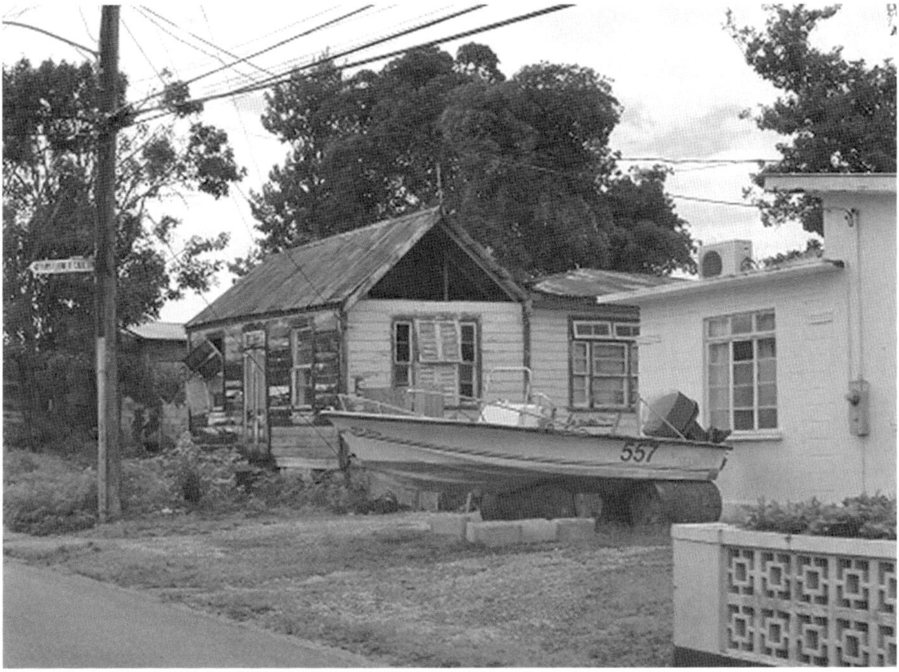
557

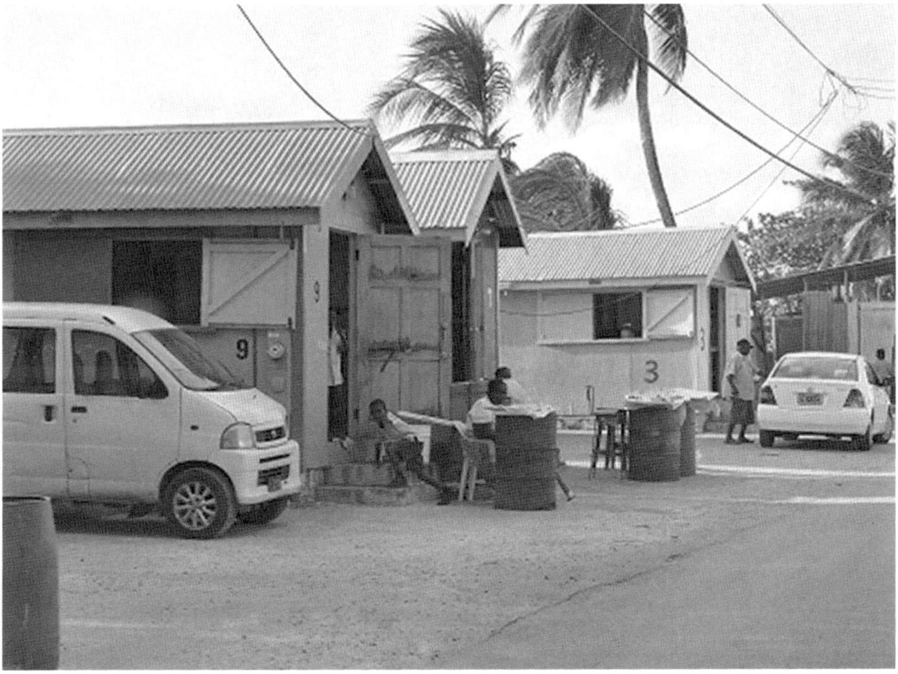
9
3

For us, these pictures call to mind, Zygmunt Bauman's notion of vagabonds and tourists. In this age of increasing globalization, all people are mobile, but both literal and virtual types of mobility are different among different peoples, with race, class, religion, and gender shaping who moves where, how they move, and whether or not they move by choice.

Plantation and Colonial Heritage

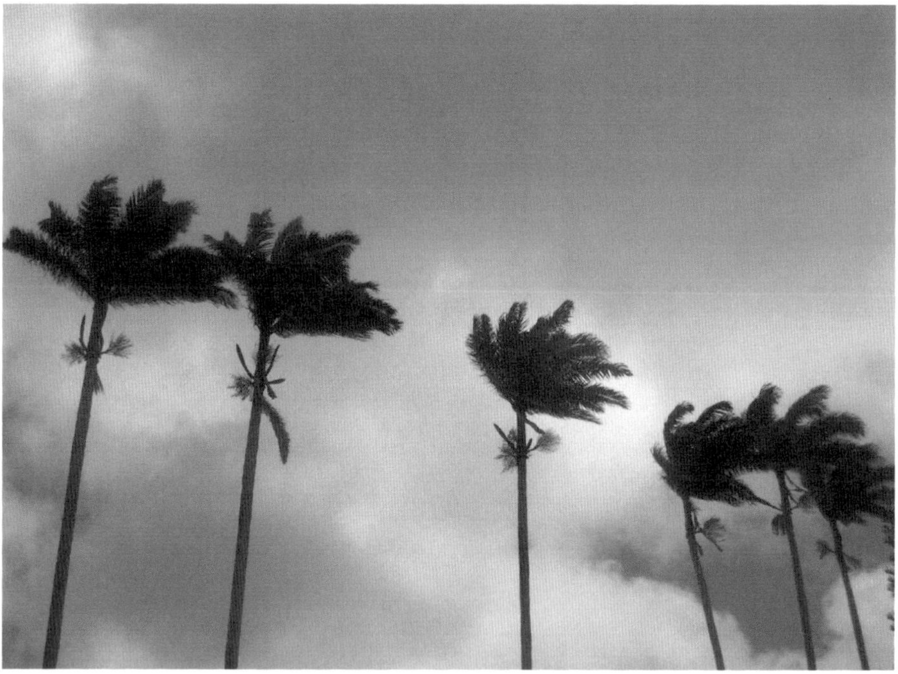

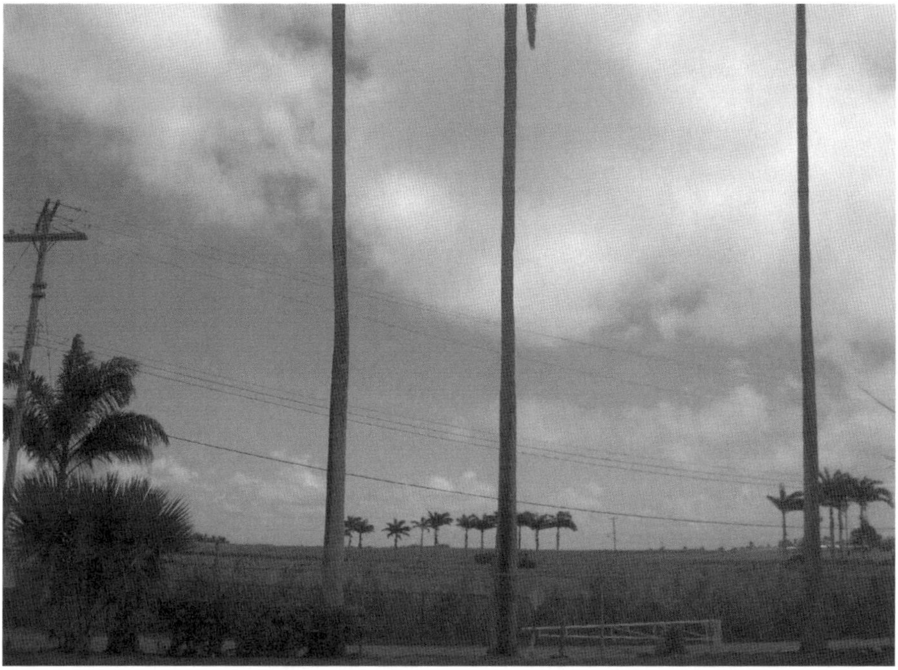

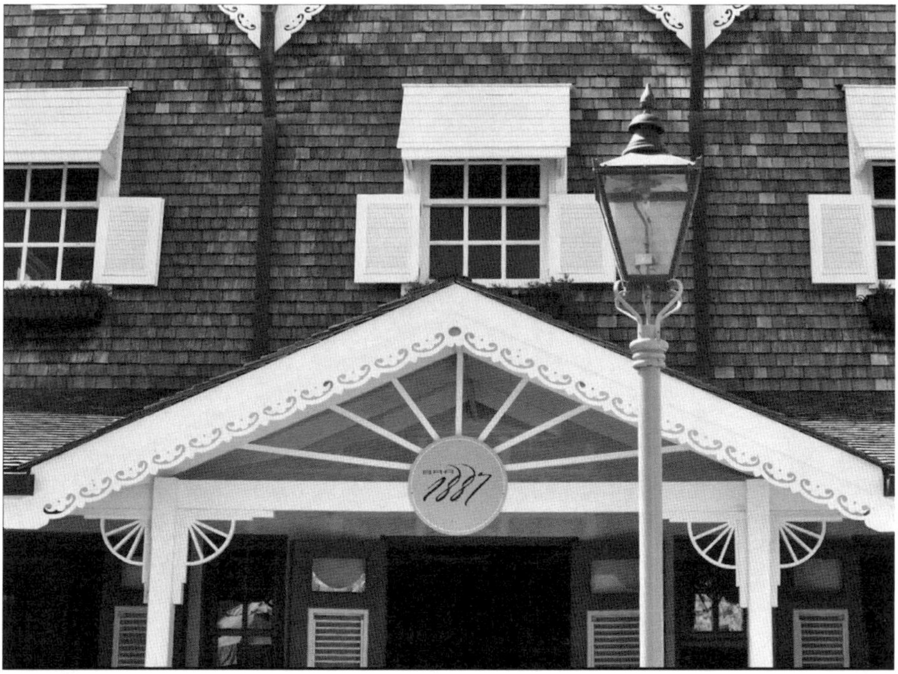
1887

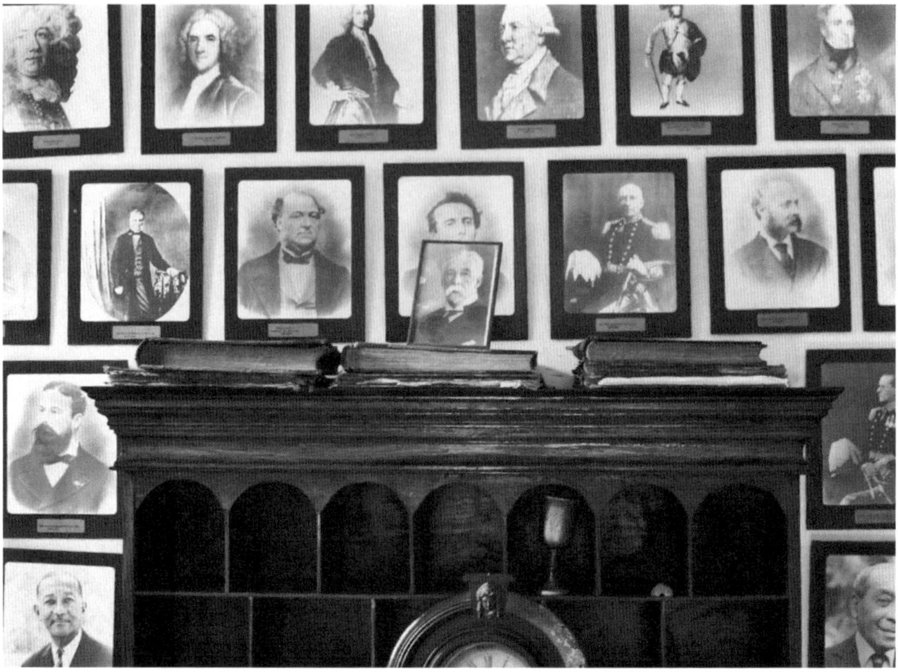

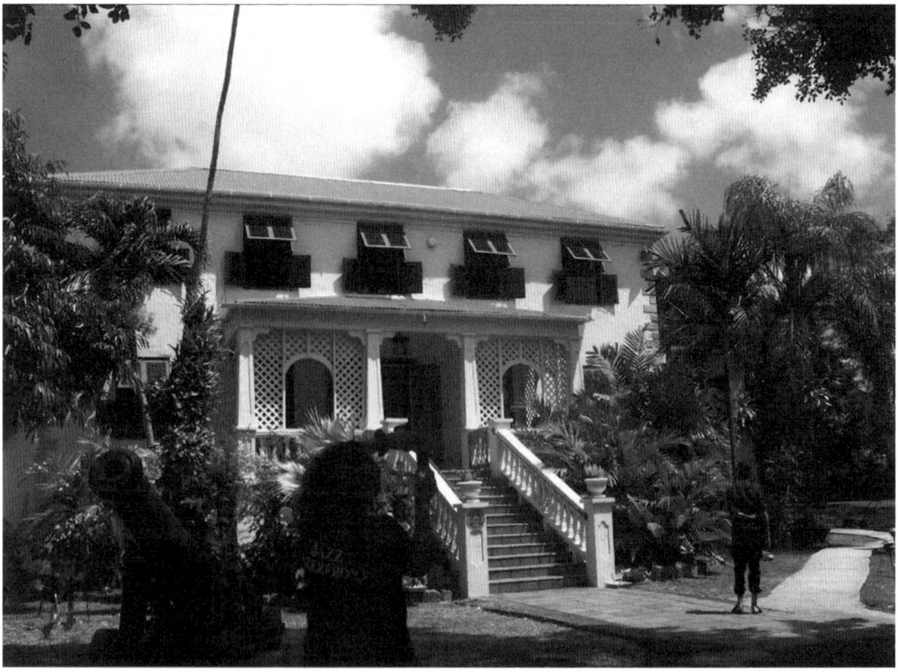

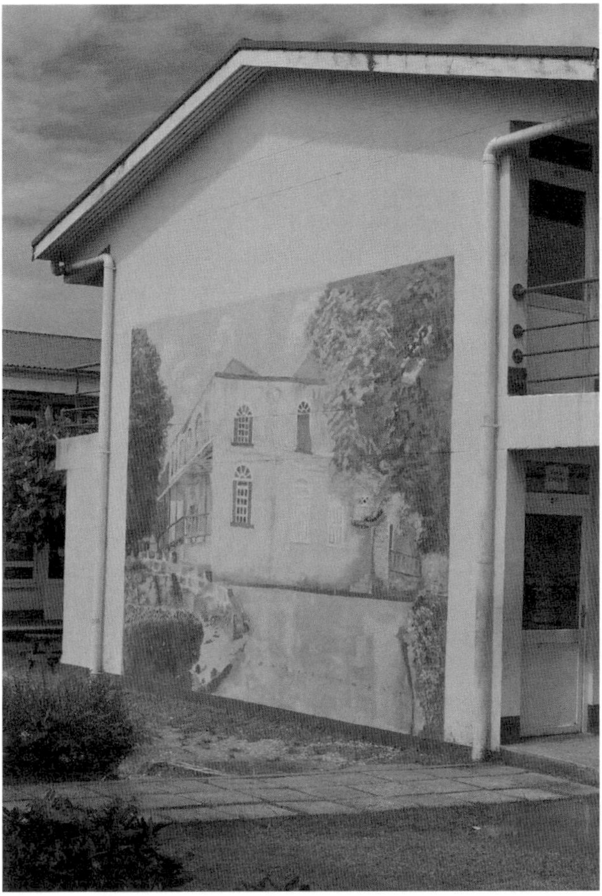

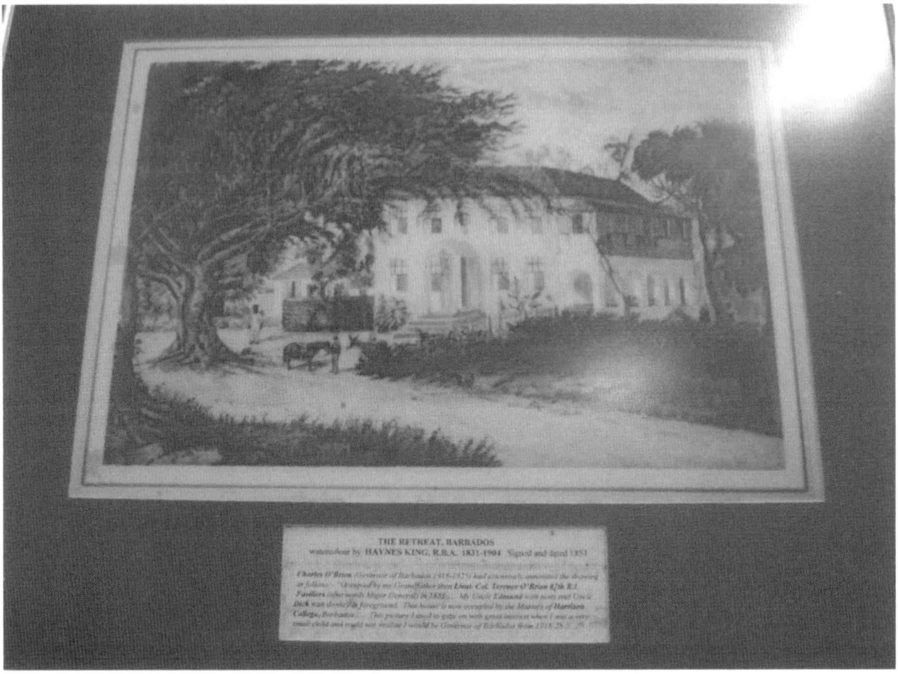
THE RETREAT, BARBADOS
watercolour by HAYNES KING, R.B.A. 1831-1904

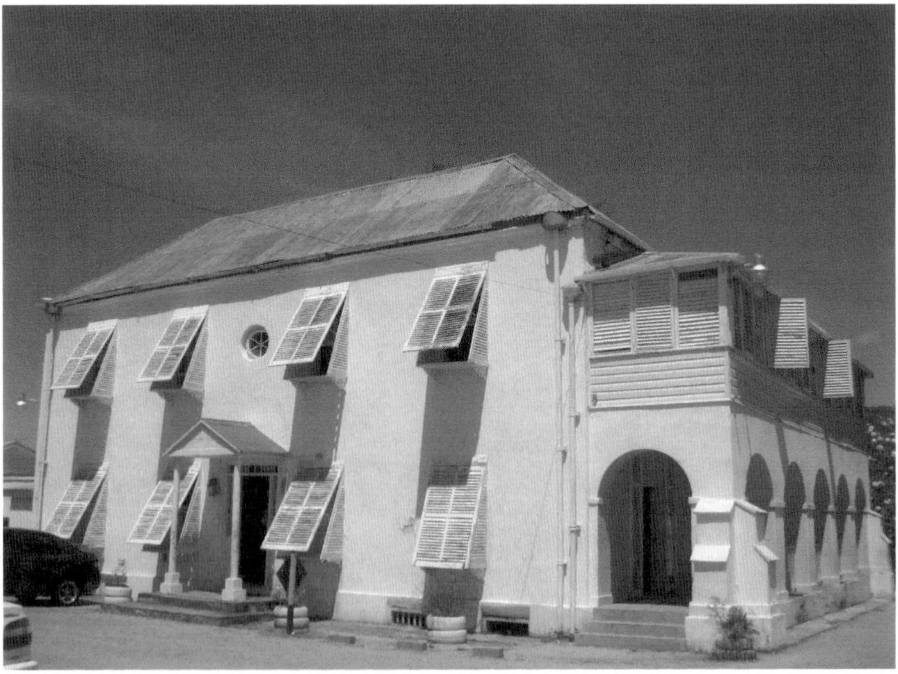

There are plantations on the island, kept and preserved as markers of the plantation past. Tourists, and school groups visit these plantations as a way of marking history. Notice the pictures on the wall of the plantation, showing the lineage of the owners. Schools are also built on the remains of plantations, and so the buildings of the school are marked and preserved as remnants of the plantation past. Notice the painting of the 'old building' now requisitioned as a school. Notice also that the Old Cloisters' staffroom was once 'The Retreat' on the plantation.

Colonial Heritage and Pageantry at Old Cloisters

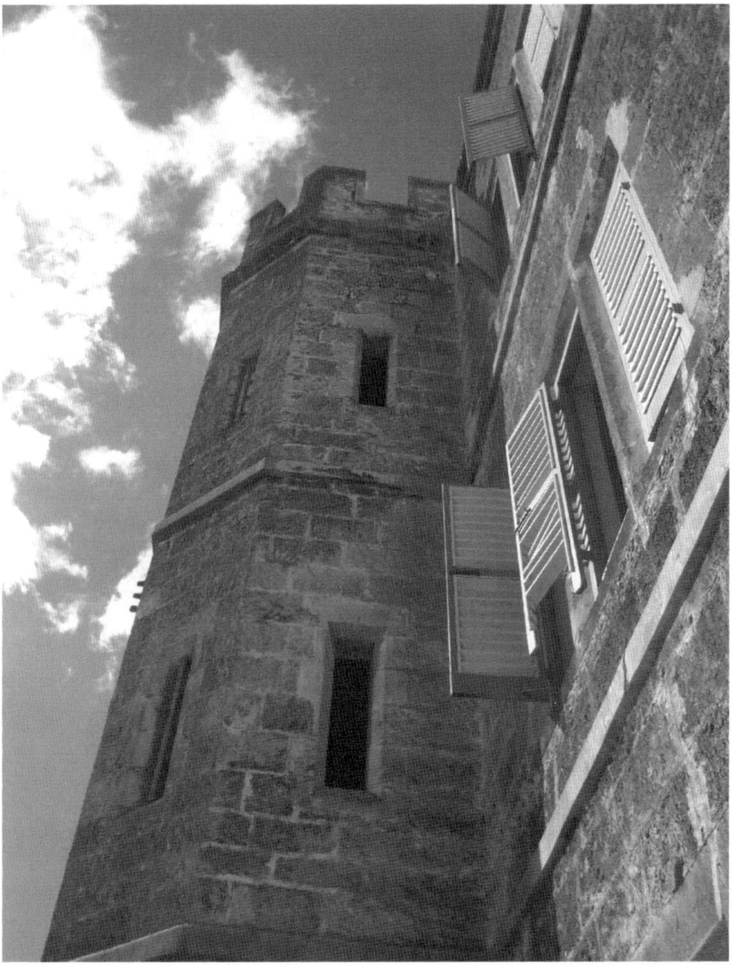

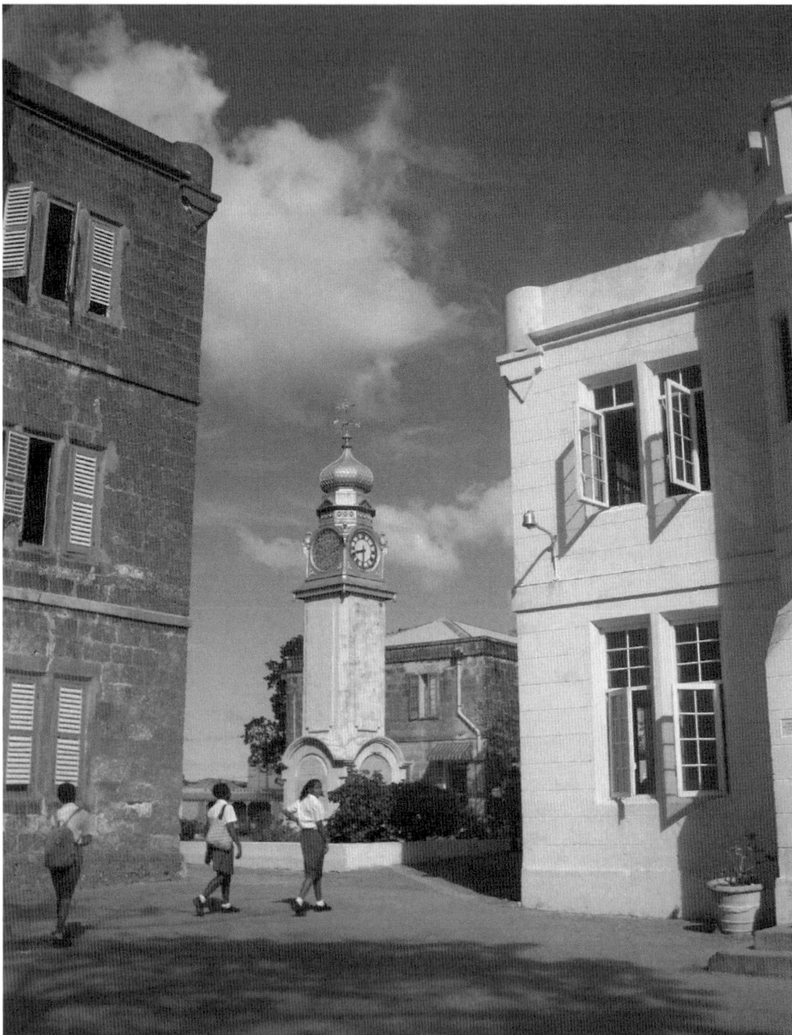

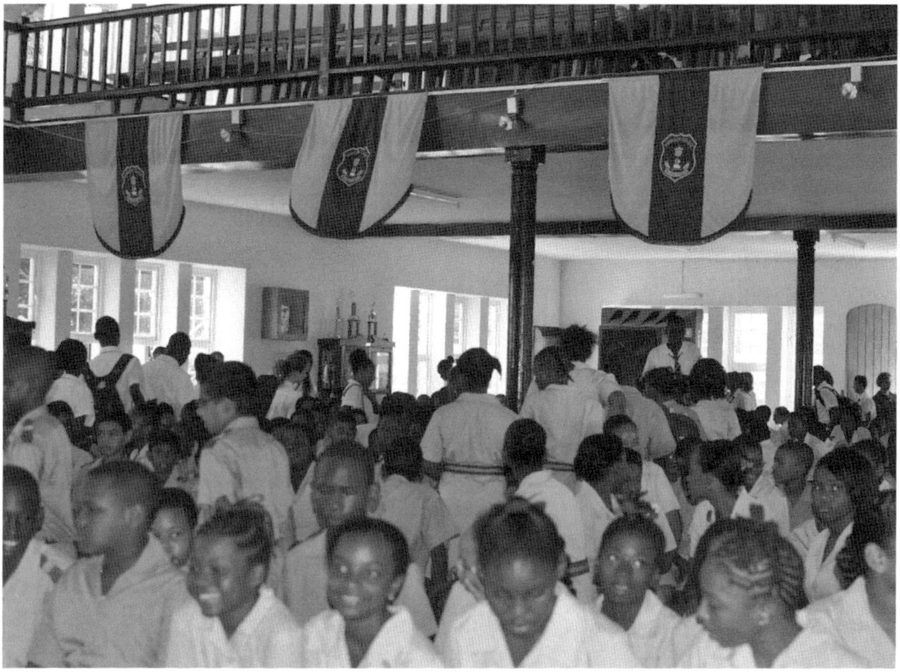

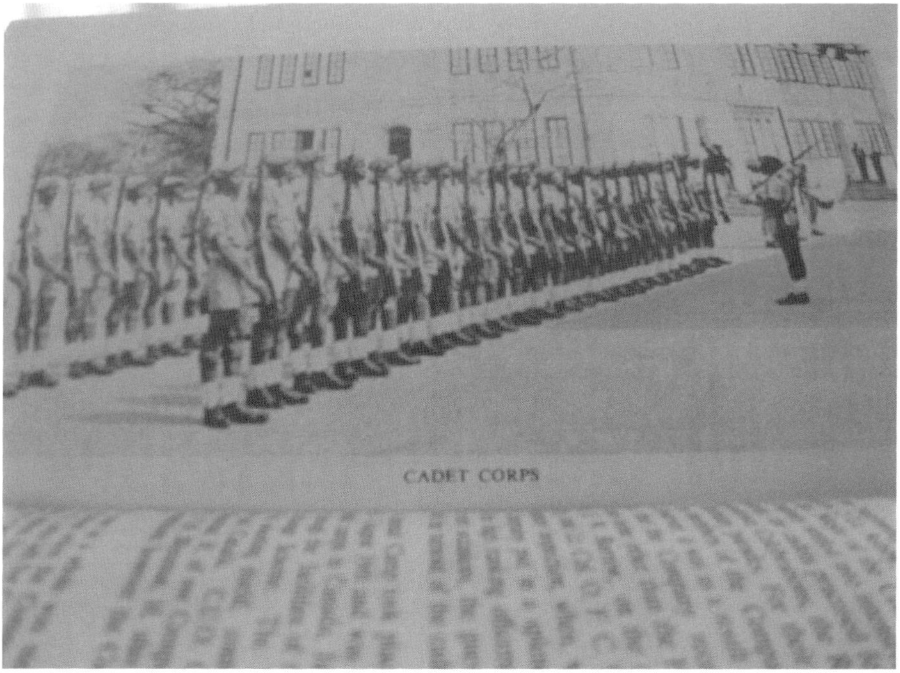
CADET CORPS

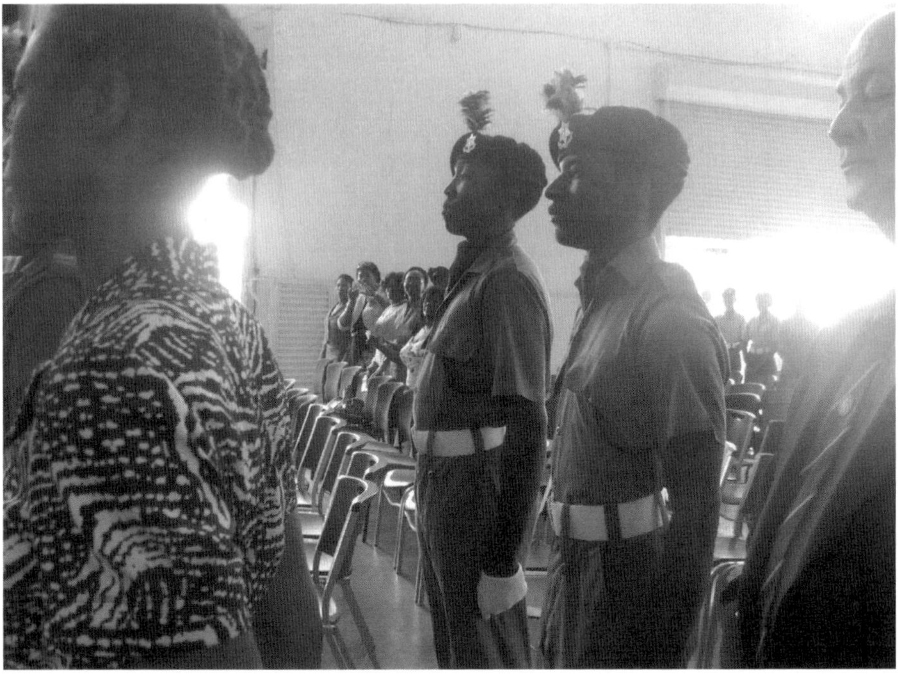

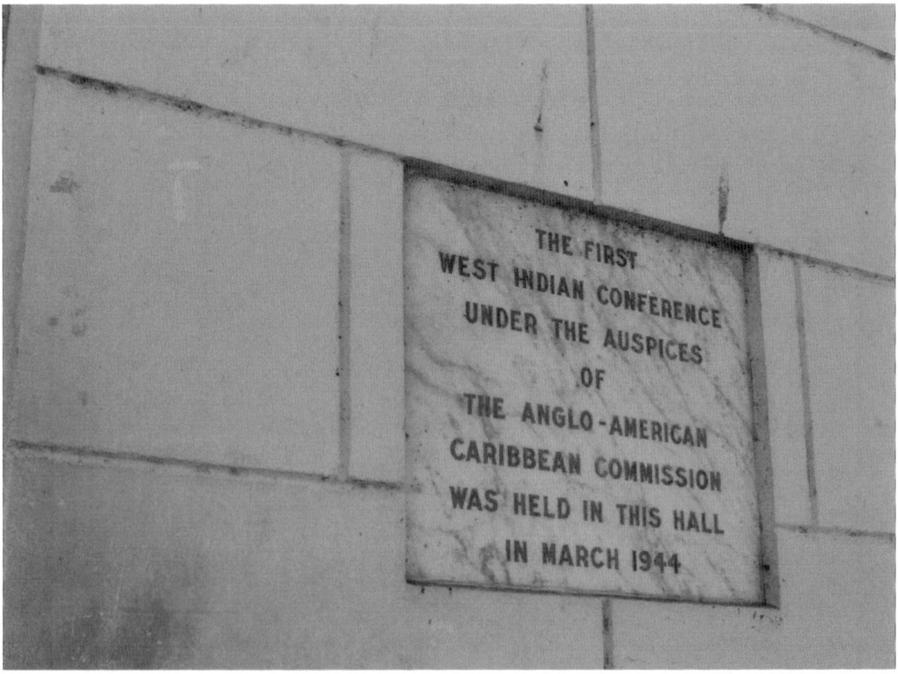
THE FIRST
WEST INDIAN CONFERENCE
UNDER THE AUSPICES
OF
THE ANGLO-AMERICAN
CARIBBEAN COMMISSION
WAS HELD IN THIS HALL
IN MARCH 1944

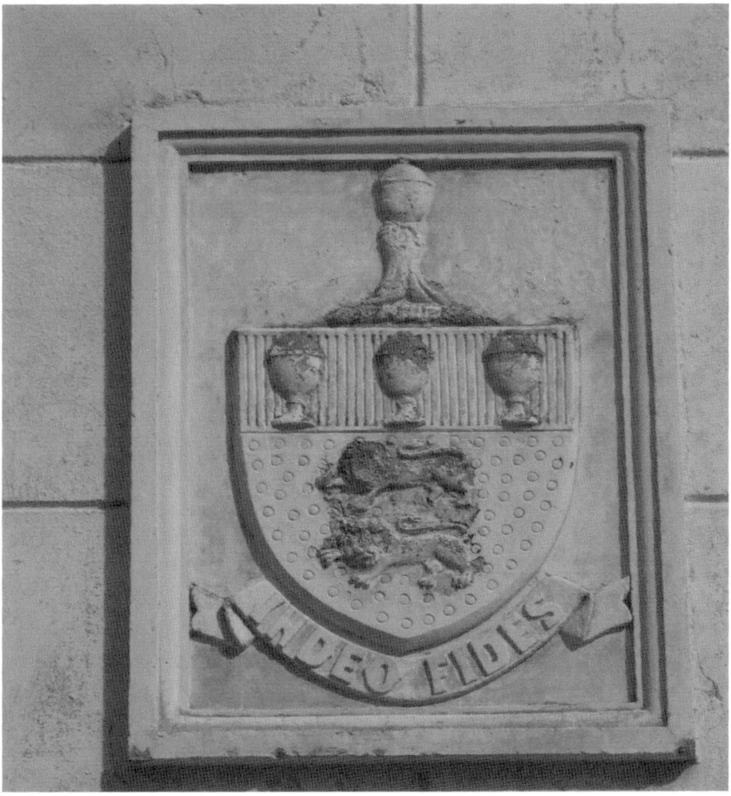
DEO FIDES

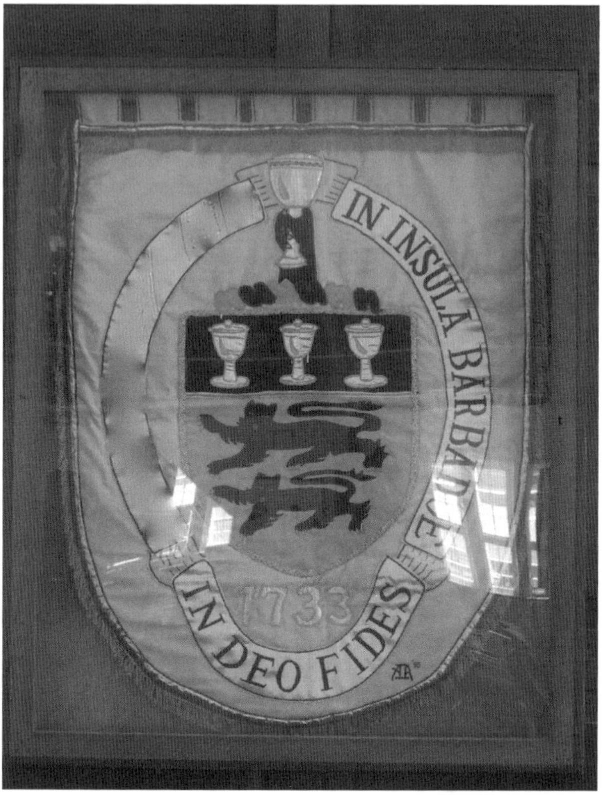

The Performance of Postcoloniality

The students engaged in a 'fashion show' where they were told to dress up in a way that would show the cultural heritage of Barbados. Notice the linkages between costuming and colonial legacies. Note, particularly, the 'Scotsman.' On the island, social class typically aligns neatly with gradient of skin color. However, there is also a class of very poor whites, descended from the Scottish people who came to Barbados as indentured servants (see Chapter "Cultivating Students' Bodies: Producing Physical, Poetic and Sociopolitical Subjectivities in Elite Schools"). We see the re-enactment of that cultural heritage by a non-white student as a sort of drag performance, with an emphasis on race not gender.

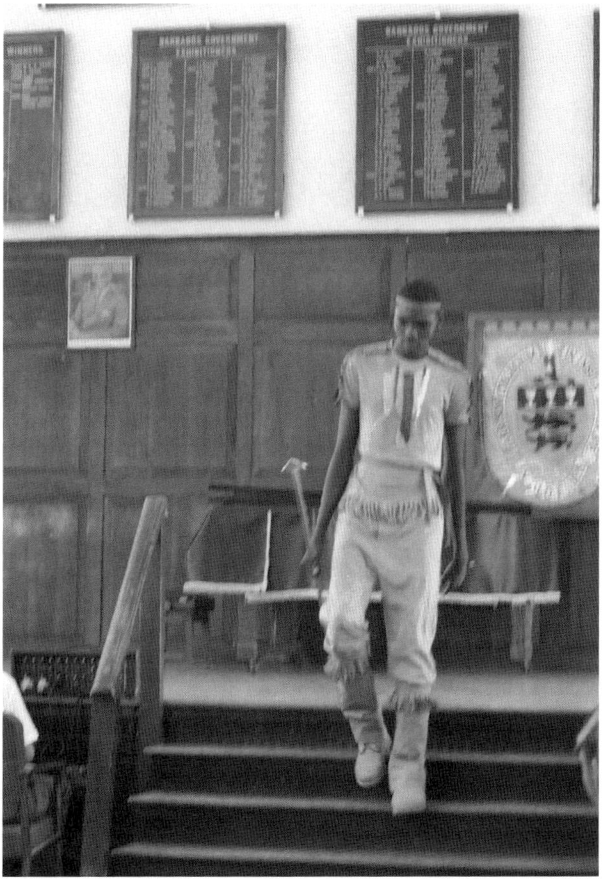

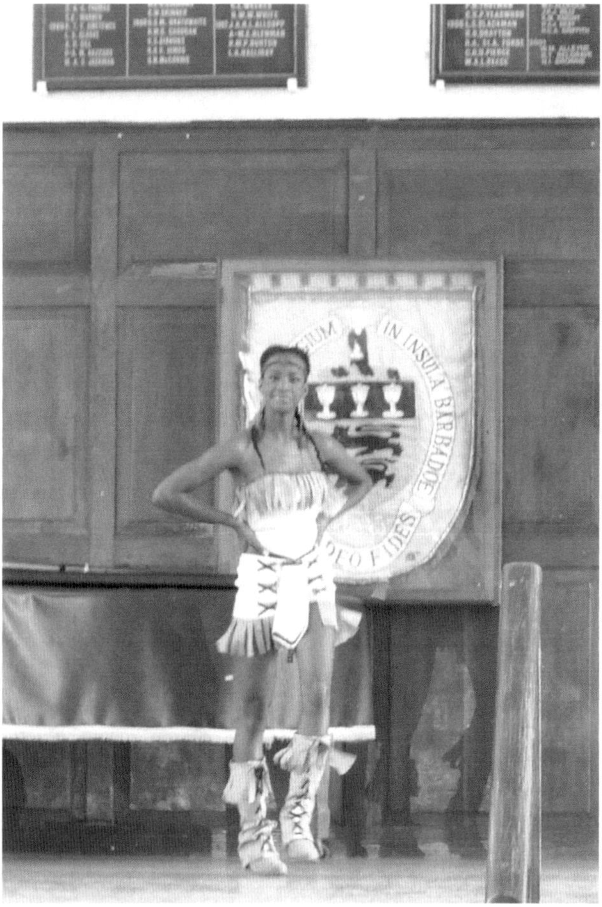
IN INSULA BARBADOE

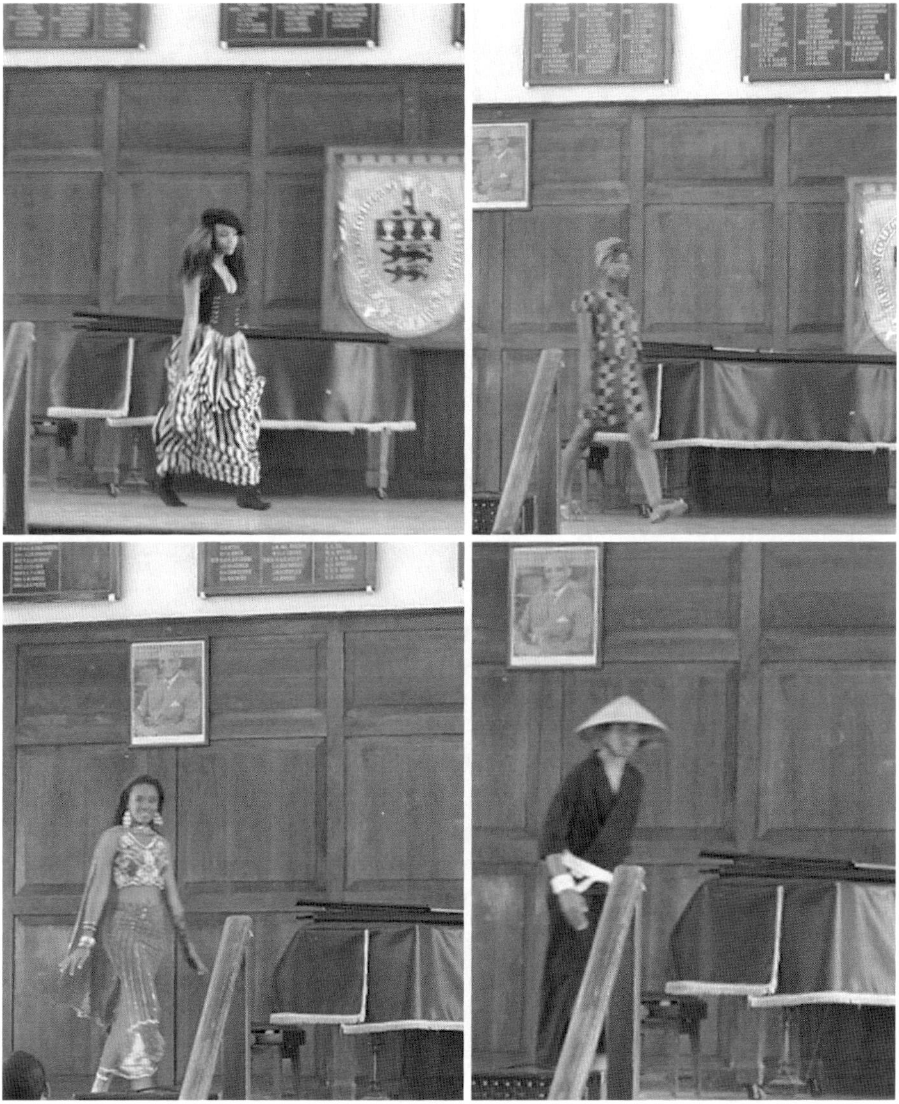

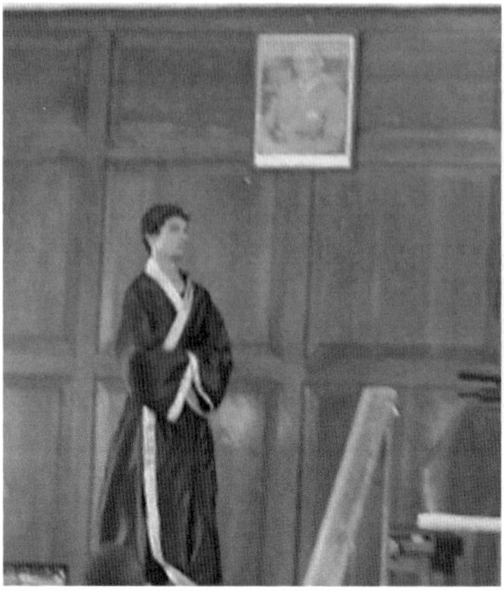

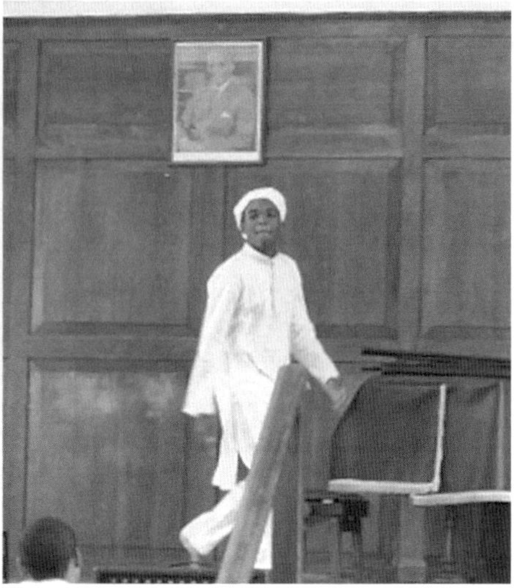

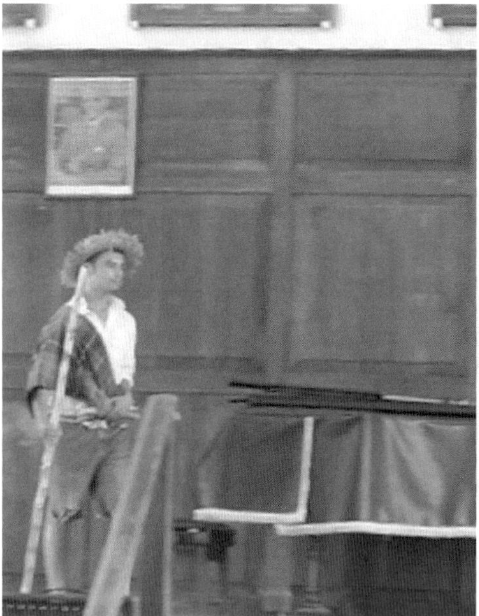

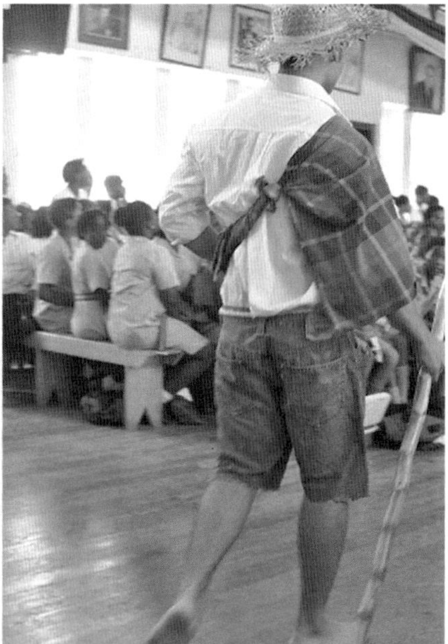

The Fashion Show Becomes both Performance and Spectacle for the Students

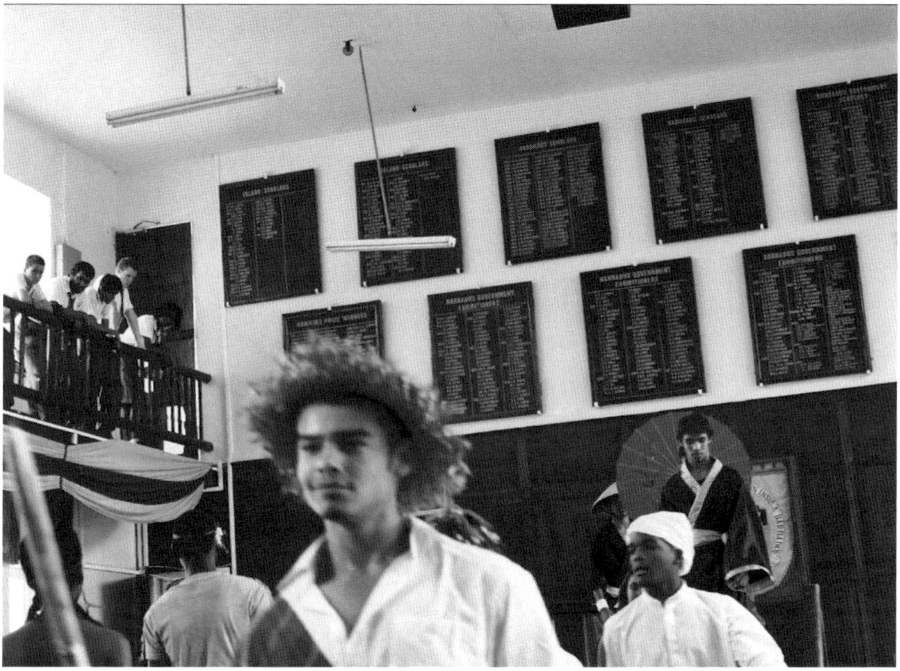

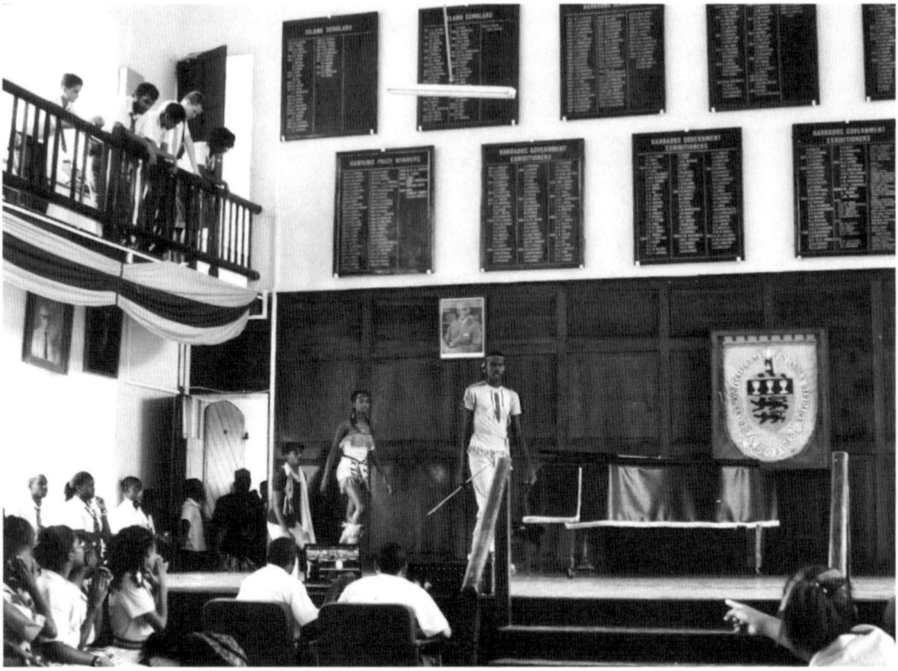

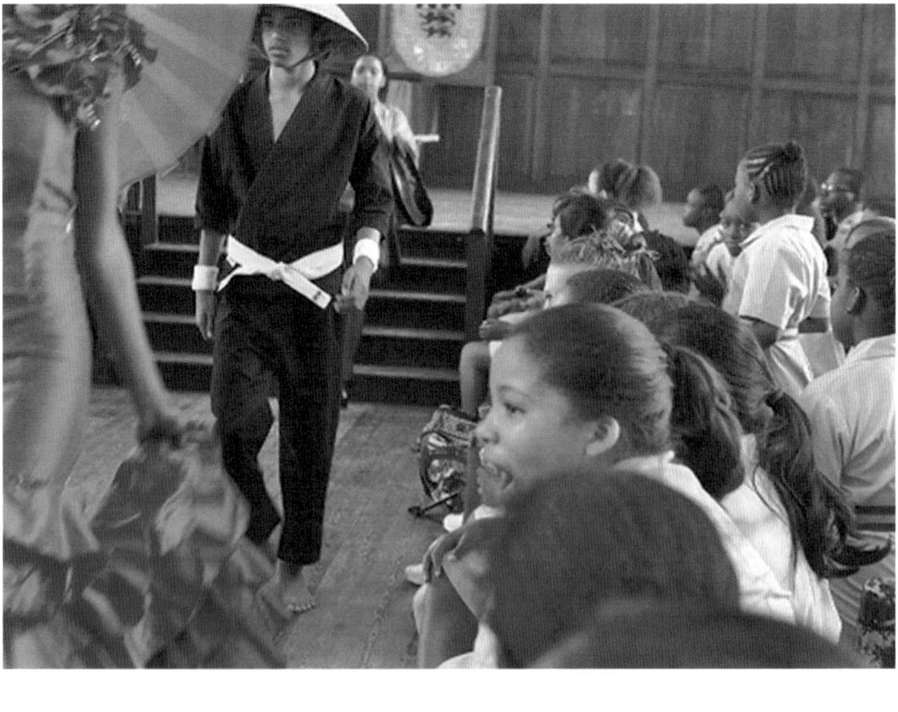

The College Fair

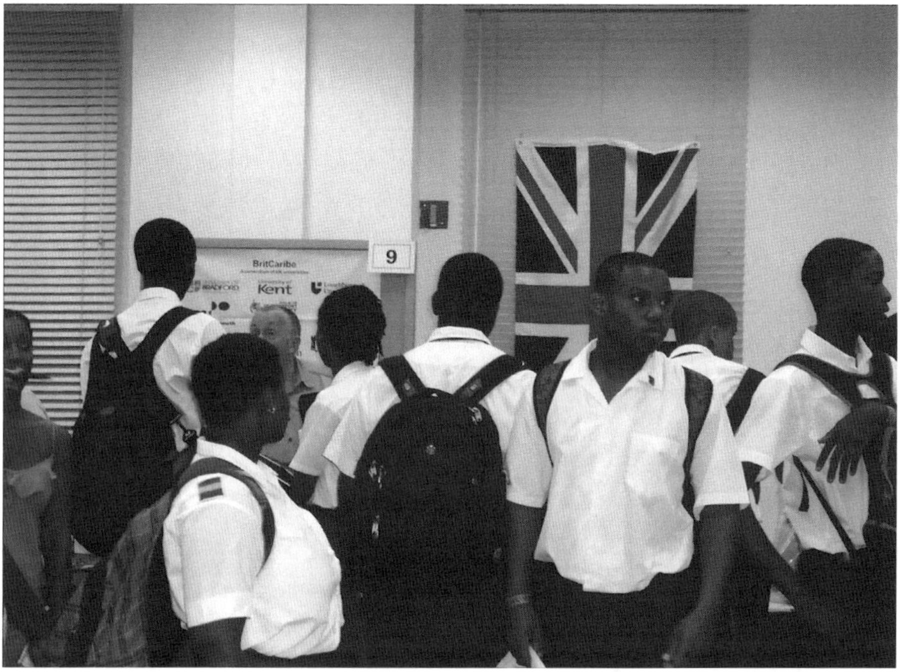

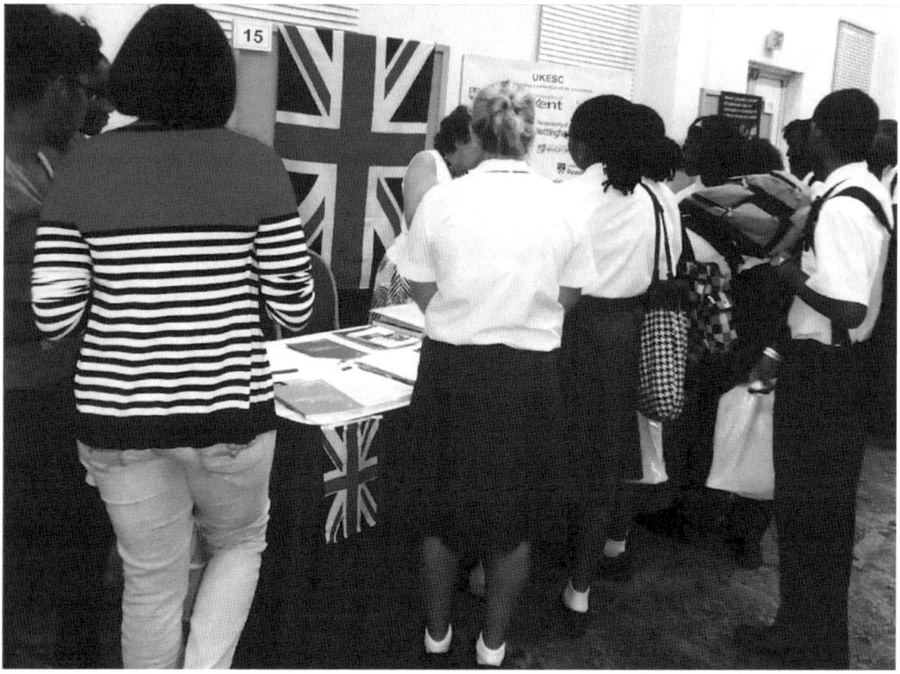

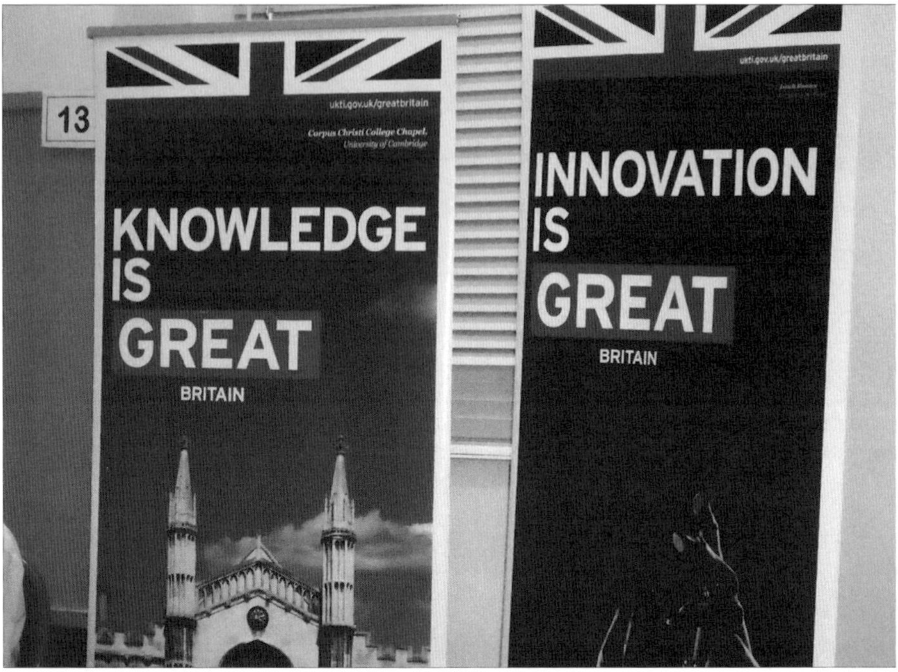
13
ukti.gov.uk/greatbritain
Corpus Christi College Chapel,
University of Cambridge
KNOWLEDGE
IS
GREAT
BRITAIN
ukti.gov.uk/greatbritain
INNOVATION
IS
GREAT
BRITAIN

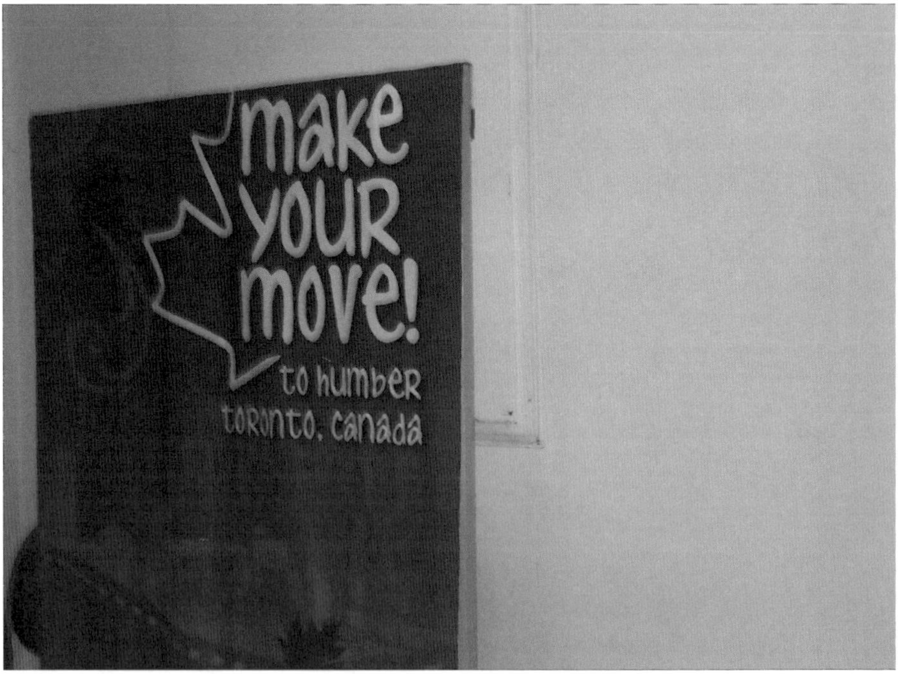
make
your
move!
to humber
toronto, canada

Concluding Remarks

In invoking and deploying PSA, we have sought to show Old Cloisters as a postcolonial school with a particularly dense language of hybridity articulated in its visual domain. This language, in the Bakhtinian (1935) sense, is 'heteroglossic.' The densely layered history of the school's past is revealed in markers in the physical environment. The aspirations of school youth manifest themselves in photographs that reveal a war of ambitions—contradictory impulses and assertions of heritage colliding with ambitions to move beyond the island to the true and only heaven in North America. Ultimately, the postcolonial school is part of a larger context in which 'histories make geographies' (Appadurai 2013, p. 61; see also Chapter "Cultivating Students' Bodies: Producing Physical, Poetic and Sociopolitical Subjectivities in Elite Schools"). The school is the harbinger of so many projects, so many dreams, so many imaginaries and imagistic landscapes! And, set as it is, in the new times of globalization and neoliberalism, it stands like Paul Klee's Angelus Novus both buoyed and buffeted by its traditions as its seeks a new parley with the present and the future.

References

Appadurai, A. (2013). How histories make geographies: Circulation and context in a global perspective. In A. Appadurai (Eds.), *The future as cultural fact: Essays on the global condition* (pp. 61–70). New York: Verso.

Bakhtin, M. (1935). Discourse in the novel. http://www.rlwclarke.net/courses/LITS3304/2008-2009/07BBakhtinDiscourseintheNovel%28Overview%29.pdf. Accessed: 31 Dec 2013.

Benjamin, W. (1968). *Theses on the philosophy of history. Illuminations* (pp. 253–264). Cambridge: The Belknap Press of Harvard University Press.

Benjamin, W. (2008). *The work of art in the age of its technological reproducibility, and other writings on Media*. Cambridge: The Belknap Press of Harvard University Press.

Berger, J. (1972). *Ways of seeing*. London: BBC and Penguin.

Bhabha, H. (1994a). *The location of culture*. New York: Routledge.

Bhabha, H. (1994b). *Sly civility. The location of culture* (pp. 93–101). New York: Routledge.

Bourdieu, P. (1993). *The field of cultural production*. New York: Columbia University Press.

Cifford, J. (1988). *The predicament of culture*. Cambridge: Harvard.

Derrida, J. (1978). *Writing and difference*. London: Routledge.

Harris, W. (1975). *Companions of the day and night*. London: Faber and Faber.

Lefebvre, H. (1992). *The production of space*. New York: Wiley-Blackwell.

Levi Strauss, D. (2003). *Between the eyes: Essays on photography and politics*. New York: Aperture.

MacDougall, D. (2006). *The corporeal image: Film, ethnography, and the senses*. Princeton: Princeton University Press.

Orwell, G. (2014). Shooting an elephant. http://www.online-literature.com/orwell/887/. Accessed: 31 Dec 2014.

Williams, A. (1983). Night and the olmec (maya series). http://www.octobergallery.co.uk/art. Accessed: 31 Dec 2013.

Cameron McCarthy Research Professor and Hardie Fellow in the Global Studies in Education Division, University of Illinois, is internationally recognized as offering unique perspectives on the politics of identity and identity of politics in contemporary education in global times. He researches intersections of race, class, gender and sexuality in theory and the classroom and has published on post-colonialism, problems with neo-Marxist writings on class, race and education, institutional support for teaching, and school rituals and adolescents. His more recent co-authored book is *New Times: Making Sense of Critical/Cultural Theory in a Digital Age* (Peter Lang 2011). Recent jointly edited books are *Mobilized Identities: Mediated Subjectivities and Cultural Crisis in the Neoliberal Era* (Common Ground 2014) and *Transnational Perspectives on Popular Culture and Public Policy: Redirecting Cultural Studies in Neoliberal Times* (Peter Lang 2008).

Heather Greenhalgh-Spencer is an assistant professor in the Department of Curriculum and Instruction at Texas Tech University. She recently finished as a visiting assistant professor in the Department of Educational Policy, Organization, and Leadership at the University of Illinois at Urbana-Champaign. Her teaching interests include global studies in education, philosophy of education, social foundations of education, and philosophy of technology. Her research interests include embodiment in online education, digital technologies as a hermeneutic for globalization, technology as global labors of production and reproduction, environmental ethics and technology, and hybrid practices of low tech/high tech educational intervention. Heather's work emerges out of scholarship in techno-feminism and techno-phenomenology. Heather's work has been published in multiple international journals, and she has received multiple scholarships in order to continue her research. She grounds both her teaching and scholarly interests in her experience as a school teacher, as a yoga teacher, and as a techno-geek.

Koeli Goel holds a PhD in Communications and Media from the University of Illinois at Urbana-Champaign and is a Post-Doctoral Research Fellow at the Institute of Communications Research, UIUC. Her work adopts a critical approach to communication and cultural studies with a focus on studying twentyfirst-century conditions of globalization especially in postcolonial societies as they are configured by new media practices, social movements and neoliberal restructuring of the state, enterprise and the individual. Her diverse research interests also include NGO engagement in public policy formulation, visual culture, elite and subaltern studies, museum studies, multicultural and critical discourse analysis, and online communities. Her abiding academic commitment through the years is also towards gender relations in international development. Her recent work has been as a member of an international group of researchers from various universities across the world studying elite education and culture across several continents like United States, Australia, Asia, Europe and South America and the Caribbean. Koeli's work has been published in journals such as *Qualitative Inquiry, Studies in Symbolic Interaction, British Journal of Sociology of Education*, and *Globalization, Societies and Education.*

Chunfeng Lin formerly a Chinese Journalism Award-winning journalist, is a Doctoral Candidate at the Institute of Communications Research at University of Illinois, Urbana-Champaign. His work centers on the issues connecting media, propaganda and space, media history, social and critical theory. His recent work on Chinese neorealist cinema has been published in the journal *Studies in the Humanities*. As a member of an international collective of researchers from seven countries investigating elite schooling in globalizing circumstances, Chunfeng's latest work has been accepted for publication by *British Journal of Sociology of Education.*

Michelle Castro is a PhD candidate in the Department of Education Policy, Organization and Leadership at the University of Illinois at Urbana-Champaign. She has worked as a bilingual teacher at elementary and university level and continues to tutor students who speak English as another language. Her interests lie in language ideology, globalization, and post-colonialism. Her dissertation work will specifically look at how compulsory language learning interplays with students' social imaginaries.

Brenda Sanya is a Ph.D. student at the University of Illinois, Urbana-Champaign. Sanya holds a dual B.A. in Philosophy & Psychology, and an interdisciplinary M.A. in Gender and Cultural Studies. Broadly, her research explores race, gender, sexuality, education, citizenship, migration and transnationalism. She interrogates formal and informal structures as spaces where gender, race and citizenship performance and performativity are produced and reproduced, and circulated in and through global landscapes. Her recent work on feminism, mobility and technology in Kenya has been published in the journal *Feminist Africa* and in *Mobilized Identities: Mediated Subjectivities and Cultural Crisis in the Neoliberal Era* (Common Ground 2014).

Ergin Bulut received his PhD from the Institute of Communications Research at the University of Illinois at Urbana Champaign. He is currently an assistant professor at the Department of Media and Visual Arts at Koc University, Turkey. His research interests cover political economy of media and media labor, critical/cultural studies, game studies, and philosophy of technology. He teaches in the following areas: globalization of culture and communication; sociology of communication and information; identity, power and people. His writings have appeared in *TV and New Media; Globalization, Societies and Education*; and *Review of Education, Pedagogy, and Cultural Studies*. He is the co-editor of *Cognitive Capitalism, Education, and Digital Labor* (Peter Lang 2011).

Vignette: Sight

Matthew Shaw

My perception of a high-achieving, fee charging school prior to arriving in Cyprus extended beyond the classroom as there was a visual appeal that dovetailed with the reputation for high achieving students. I envisioned significant amounts of green space in the form of well-tended grounds and gardens with walk-ways that were clear of clutter and well maintained. The buildings would be clean and stately, dating from the height of the imperial period with intricately carved figures on and around the sandstone or red-brick buildings—denoting a grandeur associated with the status the school seeks—and separating it visually from schools in the public sector. Internally the rooms would be comfortable, well-equipped and modern. The visual splendor and resources would be a sight for potential students to admire and aspire to learn in and a high-quality learning environment for those currently attending.

The Lefkos Academy (TLA), however, does not fit into the mold that I had created in my imagination. It is on the academic level that the school's performance and reputation attest to its elite status. The standard of the school's grounds and buildings are a different matter. In appearance, it is hard to distinguish it from other schools within Nicosia. Some staff members compared the facilities unfavorably to those they had experienced in the UK comprehensives—and that is without adding in the fees that TLA charges.

The outside of the main building looks impressive with its sandstone visage and arches running along the whole of its back side as an external corridor. This look evokes Victorian England, correlating with the period when the school was founded. However, inside the rooms, movements from other classrooms echo loudly. The temperature varies between cold in the winter and hot in the summer due to inadequate heating and air conditioning. The school's other buildings share the same problems. There are two clusters of mobile classrooms that are little more than tin boxes equipped with a whiteboard, projector and computer, air conditioner and a set of small desks and plastic chairs for the students. They were necessary, however, because another building had been knocked down because it was unsafe.

There is also a sports precinct on the eastern side of the campus at the bottom of the hill. It includes an indoor gym with a multipurpose court and a football pitch

M. Shaw (✉)
Monash University, Melbourne, Australia
e-mail: matthew.shaw@monash.edu

J. Fahey et al. (eds.), *In the Realm of the Senses*, Cultural Studies and Transdisciplinarity in Education, DOI 10.1007/978-981-287-350-7_11

surrounded by an athletics track. The pitch and track are both made of gravel, red for the track, green for the pitch. There are two basketball courts, made of bitumen that is starting to crack, and three tennis courts. In addition, the school has synthetic surfaces for hockey and futsal that are in good condition.

There does not seem to be a great deal of landscaping in any part of the school's grounds apart from the garden on the eastern edge of the main building and the overall appearance of the grounds are scruffy. There are areas of untended bushland with clumps of trees—and those to the north and west of the sport center only seem to have been used to dump rubbish. Elsewhere is open tracts of land which is either overgrown or dusty depending on whether it has rained much or not. The majority of the grounds are this type of unused woodland or are open areas. These tracts of land are not utilized and are unlandscaped.

In the case of TLA, therefore, its high status within the Cypriot Community is not derived from the visage of its facilities and grounds in any way. Rather, its reputation is derived from exam results and the university destinations of its graduates, as well as the number of prospective students trying to gain admission to enjoy the academic advantage that attending the school offers. Ultimately then, the student body represents the eliteness of the school since it carries and enhances its reputation through each individuals work, brain and body.

Matthew Shaw is a PhD candidate in the Education Faculty at Monash University, Melbourne. His interests lie in history including the history of sport as well as the place of sport in schools and society. His dissertation looks at the role sport has in a divided society and the way it is used to reinforce or break down boundaries.

Looking Inside and Out: Social Aesthetics of an Elite School in India

Fazal Rizvi

Introduction

MacDougall has written extensively on the idea of social aesthetics, focusing on aesthetic systems of communities and everyday life. His work however extends well beyond written texts. He is an ethnographic filmmaker, who regards visual anthropology, vernacular photography and documentary cinema as essential tools for capturing the social aesthetics of institutions. He has also made a large number of films on indigenous communities in Australia, the life of semi-nomadic camel herders in Kenya, and various marginalized social groups in India.

My own interest in McDougall's work is not focused so much on his attempts to interpret experiences of marginalization in India but on his efforts to understand the contemporary manifestations of privilege in an elite Indian boarding school. Between 1997 and 2004, McDougall conducted a study of the prestigious Doon School in Northern India, established in the 1930s to provide education to the sons of British expatriates and the Indian ruling class. This study resulted in five films: *Doon School Chronicles* (2000), *With Morning Hearts* (2001), *Karam in Jaipur* (2001), *The New Boys* (2003), and *The Age of Reason* (2004), as well as a number of important articles on the social aesthetics of the Doon school and the possibilities of visual ethnography. These films chronicle the everyday practices of living and learning at the Doon School, highlighting not only the material but also the affective.

This work is of enormous importance to me because I too have been engaged over the past 4 years in conducting an ethnography of an elite school in India, as part of a broader international project upon which the chapters included in this collection are based. As stated earlier, this project is designed to examine the ways in

F. Rizvi (✉)
The University of Melbourne, Melbourne, Australia
e-mail: frizvi@unimelb.edu.au

J. Fahey et al. (eds.), *In the Realm of the Senses*, Cultural Studies and Transdisciplinarity in Education, DOI 10.1007/978-981-287-350-7_12

which elite schools based on the British public schools tradition in nine different countries interpret and negotiate the pressures and opportunities associated with the contemporary processes of globalization. The project has not only focused on the formal aspects of the life of these schools, such as their governance and curricular practices, but also on the social objects and sensibilities that set them apart from other schools—their markers of privilege and distinction.

One of these nine schools is in Central India: Ripon College, established in 1882 by the local Indian aristocracy to provide their sons with an education that would enable them to deal strategically and effectively with the colonial authorities. The main aim of the College was to develop in students a particular way of seeing and relating to the world, derived equally from the British and local elite traditions. Over the years, Ripon College has experienced major social, economic and cultural shifts, requiring it to negotiate not only the forces of colonialism but also postcolonial nationalism and more recently globalization. It is now a large co-educational school, struggling to preserve its elite status by retaining its colonial legacy, while, at the same, globalizing the educational outlook of its students.

MacDougall's work at the Doon School provides me with an interesting and relevant point of reference and contrast. In ways that are similar to MacDougall, I too am interested in how the social aesthetics of Ripon College is constituted; how the various landmarks on its campus generate a sense of 'sensory patterning'; and how this patterning has both affective and aesthetic dimensions that are socially structured. However, unlike MacDougall who provides a portrayal of the social aesthetics of the Doon School, I am also interested in exploring Ripon College's social aesthetics in order to understand how it generates and distributes its sense of privilege among its students, parents and teachers. I want to argue that the social aesthetics of Ripon College is a product not only of what lies and is enacted within the school but also how its interior is linked to what lies beyond its borders—in the local and national communities as well as the global context in which the College is now seeking to locate itself.

MacDougall on Social Aesthetics

As has been noted in the Introduction to this collection, MacDougall articulates his idea of social aesthetics in direct opposition to the traditional notions of aesthetics, conceptualized in popular parlance as a matter of taste, concerned primarily with the appreciation of beauty in art and nature, involving a set of value judgments. In the Western traditions, this view is based largely on the Enlightenment ideas relating to the singularity of the self. It involves a critical elaboration of the manner in which individuals engage with art and object. For MacDougall, the idea of social aesthetics is much broader, and involves a wider range of social interactions relating to 'culturally patterned sensory perceptions' (MacDougall 2006, p. 94). In this sense, aesthetic experience is more experimental than simply a cognitive engagement with a work of art. It is not arbitrary or random, but is socially configured, structured around a variety of culturally defined meanings. Social aesthetics, for MacDougall, thus refers to a set of interactions between sense impressions and social practices.

Traditionally, the study of aesthetics involved attempts to describe the manner in which artists in particular attempt to intervene in social structures and values through the creation of objects, performance or situations that challenged these structures. MacDougall, in contrast, views social aesthetics as a term that can be used beyond the parameters of any distinct art form towards a new understanding of aesthetics that is fundamentally concerned with the relationships of people to people and the framing of these relationships in ways that maintain and challenge these social values and structures. This social sense of aesthetics is thus linked to relations of sociality, involving both 'cognitive' and 'affective' dimensions. The study of aesthetics can thus be approached not only with respect to objects of art but also everyday practices. In this way, MacDougall views social aesthetics as a rediscovery of aesthetics in the everyday.

In line with this thinking, MacDougall's visual portrayal of the Doon School is designed to highlight sensory patterning of the school's everyday activities. It is based on a view that the culture of the Doon School is in a large part mediated through the sensuous. In his portrayal of the school, MacDougall is not so much interested in assessing the beauty of the campus but in showing how it is through the senses that the qualities of its environment (dominant patterns of color, texture, movement and behavior) should be interpreted. He maintains that although 'aspects of material culture have always constituted a major topic for anthropology, these tended to disappear within larger questions of belief and social structure' (MacDougall 2008, p. 6).

Through visual anthropology, MacDougall insists, social aesthetics can be shown to be both ubiquitous and yet highly dispersed through a wide range of cultural phenomena. It needs to be accessed indirectly through various visual, aural, verbal, temporal and tactile domains. MacDougall's films are designed to access these domains, in an attempt to interpret the sensory patterns that constitute the Doon School's everyday cultural practices. Without the benefit of films, in this essay, I want to focus on a number of Ripon College's key sites as a way of showing how they help to structure sensory patterning at the College, and how its social aesthetics plays a crucial role in defining and normalizing its elite status.

The Main Building

Ripon College was established in 1882 in Central India for the education of the boys of the local aristocracy—the Maharajas, Rajkumars and Nawabs. The regional British political agent in central India, after whom the school is named, viewed the creation of the College as an initiative designed to provide the sons of the local aristocracy a distinctively English education. The key aim of the College was to initiate its students into English attitudes and cultural dispositions. In this sense, the creation of Ripon College involved a political accommodation of a sort through which British and local elite interests were both realized. The local aristocracy thus funded the development of the College, even as the responsibility for its management was left to the colonial administrators.

In its organizational structure, Ripon College was modeled in the image of a number of other schools created by the colonial authorities earlier for the Indian aristocracy, such as Mayo College in Ajmer, established in 1869. Like Mayo, Ripon College viewed itself as a symbol of a progressive modern culture. It proclaimed the dawn of a new enlightened age, an imagined future that was assumed to be accessible only to Indian princes, who were believed to have had the capacity to access higher civilizations in ways other Indian communities could not. The 'lesser communities' had to be led by them; the Indian aristocratic class was believed to have had the capacity to interpret and translate for other Indians the still superior English cultural norms, practices and institutions. In this way, Ripon College, from its very beginning, had assumed for itself an elite status.

Ripon College elite status was further enhanced when, in the early 1900s, it received a donation of nearly 120 acres of land from the local aristocracy, in 'anticipation of a brighter future'. Boarding houses were built on this land in the image of British public schools, structured in ways that enabled the masters to maintain routine and discipline. However, it was the main building of the school, which had many similarities with Mayo College, which set the College apart from the rest of the city in which it was located. Sanjay Srivastava (1998, p. 44) has shown how in a number of ways the architectural style of Mayo College's main building expresses an ideological form that displays 'its historical grandeur, its genuflection towards an 'Otherness', as well as its progressive aspirations couched in terms of the colonial sense of cultural superiority'.

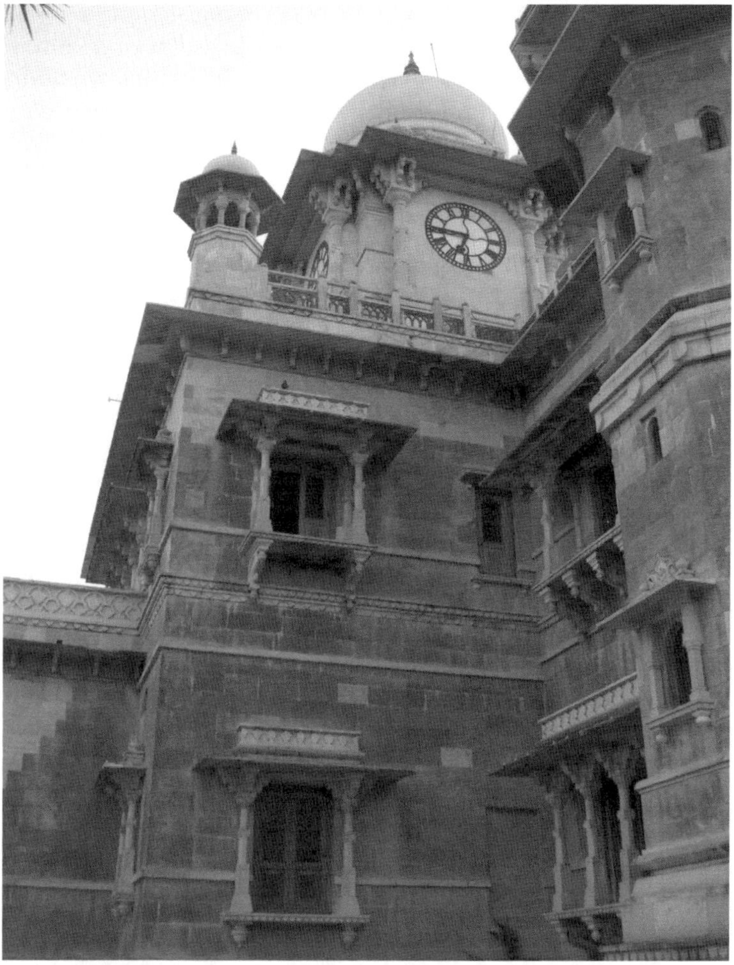

Like Mayo College, the main building of Ripon is also constructed from white marble, and is adorned with numerous canopies, minarets and arches in the Indo-Saracenic style. Its grandeur is deliberately incongruous with its surroundings, designed to highlight its elite status as an institution that reflects its glorious Oriental past, while at the same time symbolizing historical progress. Like Mayo College, the main building of Ripon College has a large clock, symbolizing progress, modernity, rationality and order. According to Srivastava (1998, p. 46), in colonial India, the clock towers expressed a system of meaning that was constituted by a "discursive universe of nineteen century Europe; a world which perceived its difference from the ethos of Oriental existence through the intellectual and spiritual elaborations of the European Renaissance and through the mechanisms of the industrial revolution". Srivastava adds that, "clock towers marked, both literally and symbolically, the route the native might take to the realms of modernity".

For both Mayo and Ripon Colleges, this route became the very reason for their existence. The clock symbolized the journey the students must take towards progress in order to provide leadership to the rest of the Indian community. Today, the main building stands proudly in the middle of the campus, surrounded by beautifully landscaped gardens. The visitors to the College are left in no doubt that they are approaching a place of considerable importance. In advertising the College on its websites and other media, long shots of the building are used to represent Ripon College as a 'heritage school'. Pointing to its authoritative importance, the Principal's office is in the middle of building. It is surrounded by classrooms for senior students, where they are expected to be quite and deferential. The students and teachers alike readily accept this sensory patterning: they behave in the main building in ways in which they might not in other parts of the College.

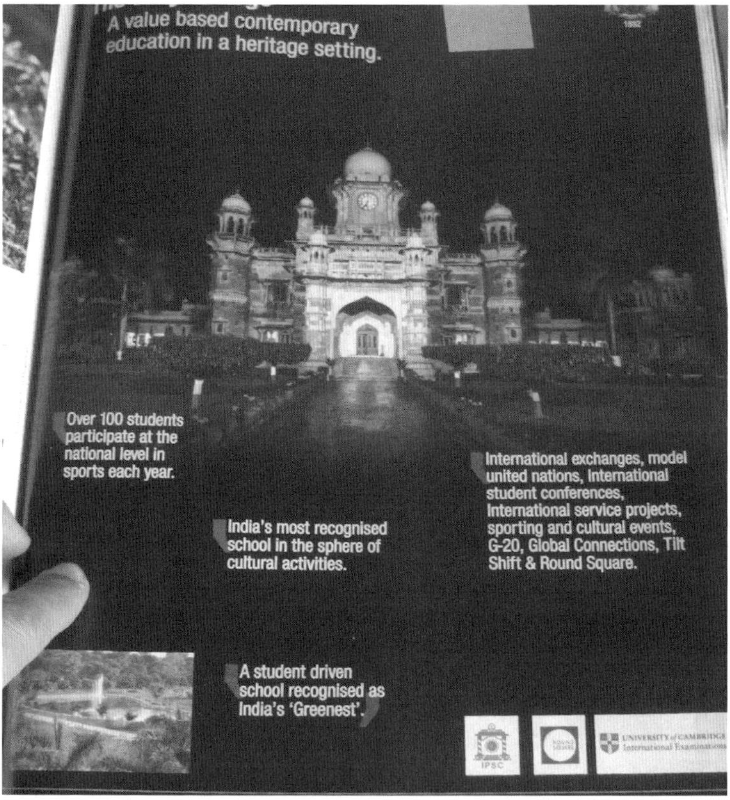

Until 2008, the main building incorporated an assembly hall, which was used for most school-wide functions, such as orientation, graduation, teacher workshops and of course school assembly at the beginning of each day. When a new large auditorium, funded by a major Indian philanthropist, was built in 2007, the assembly hall was converted into an elaborate meeting room for major ceremonial occasions. The Board of Governors now uses it for its meetings and functions. The hall is now decked out with old furniture, large paintings of the College's original donors and various other museum pieces. For most students, if the sensory experience of the old assembly hall were not daunting enough, the new meeting room, now named, somewhat grandly, as the 'darbar' [a royal court], has become prohibitively exclusive. It is almost invariably locked, and the students view it as a special space which is accessible only to a very few. They aspire to be allowed in.

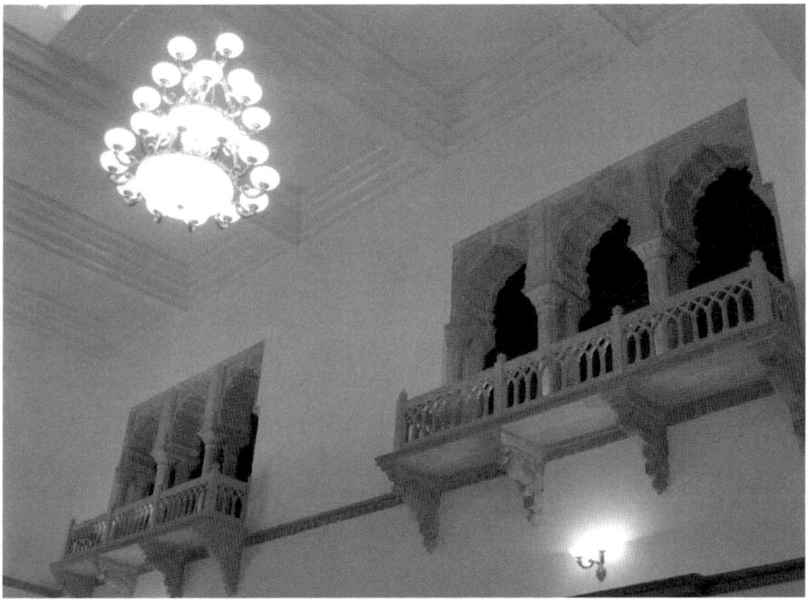

The Gate

In the late 1990s, another symbol of prestige was erected at Ripon College. With financial support from an alumnus of the College, who had become a major businessman in India, the College replaced the wooden gate to its sprawling campus with a tall brick structure, in the image of a gate to palaces. The gate was never intended to serve a security function, as the old gate performed a perfectly acceptable role in marking the College's boundaries. Instead it acquired many other functions. Most significantly, according to the College's Estate Manager, the gate is designed to instill in students a sense of pride: 'to recognize that they are at a special place'. The gate has been named 'Gyan Dwar', a Hindi word that means gate to knowledge. Once they pass through the gate, the students are expected to realize that they have been permitted into a zone of privilege not accessible to most other Indians. The gate is constructed to communicate a particular understanding of knowledge, as inextricably linked to modalities of power. This understanding is not described, but rather is based on a relation between materiality and affect, the idea that 'things' can evoke particular feelings in a whole range of non-representational ways within social aesthetics.

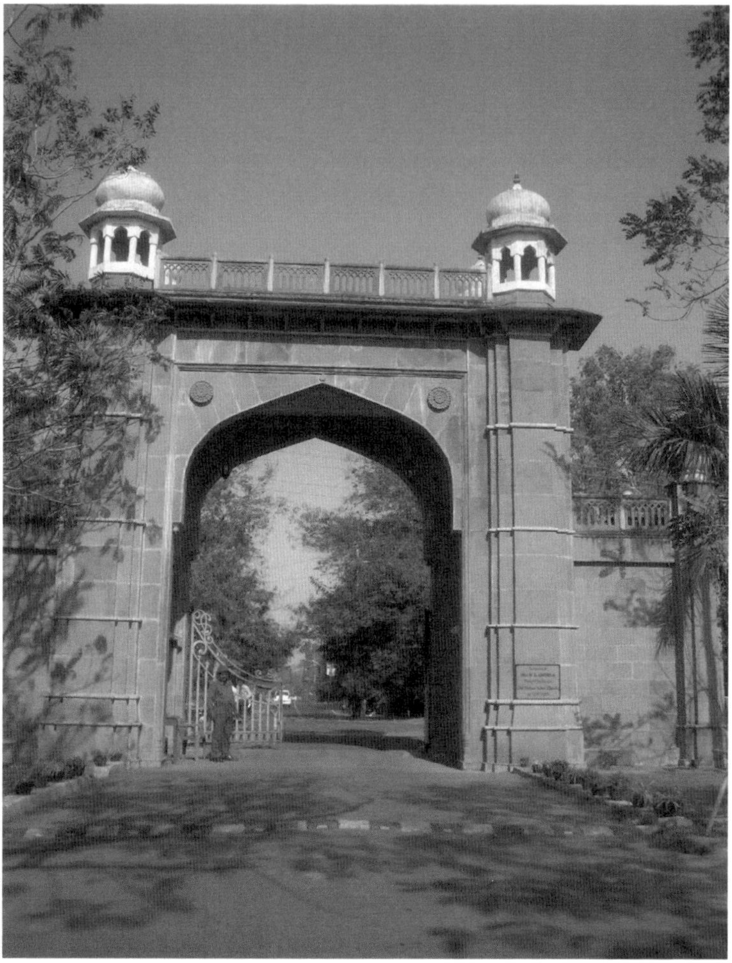

The students readily accept the significance of the gate. According to an alumni who was a student when the gate was built, and still lives in the city where Ripon College is located, "the gate gave us confidence. When you passed the gate, you got a surge of pride…you felt important, that you were entering a place that is something great". According to the current students too the gate is a major signifier of the College's social standing in the city. 'When I come into the school in the morning, I can see it from a kilometer away, and I know I am going to somewhere special', said a student, adding that the gate helped her organize her thoughts for the day. To other students, the gate represents an entry into a place that is spacious, tidy and attractive, in a marked contrast to what lies outside the campus.

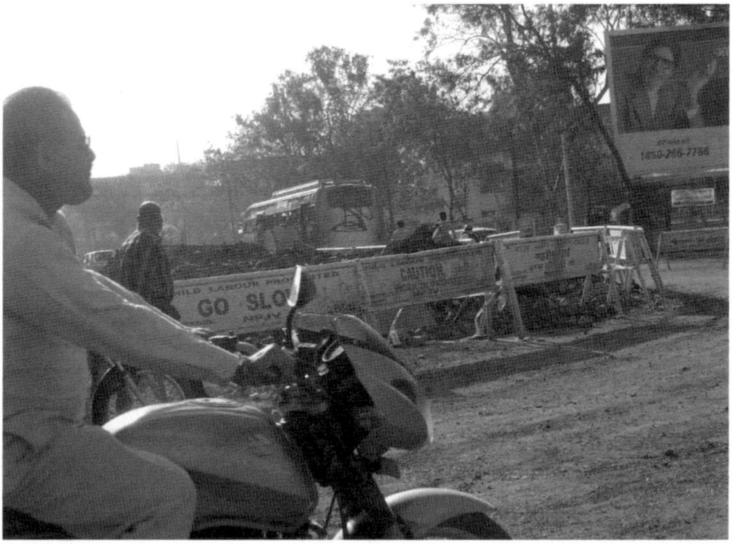

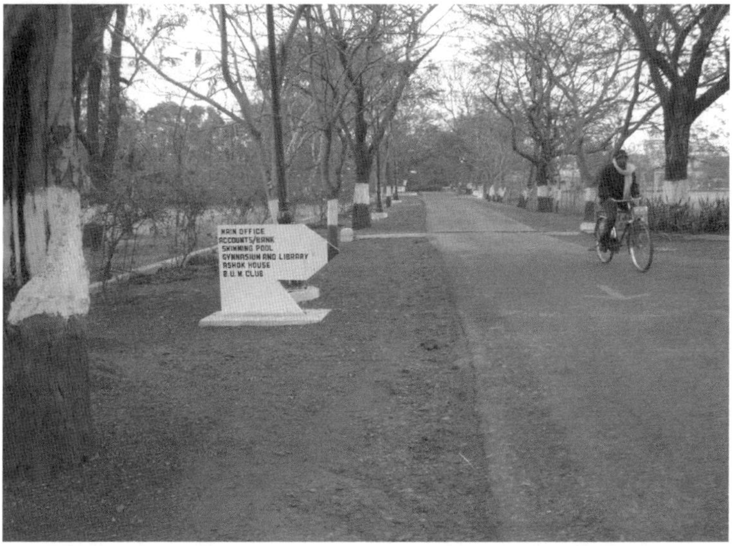

Some very poor communities surround Ripon College's campus, resulting from migration from the nearby villages to the city. Even by local standards, the streets are a great deal more crowded, dusty and dirty, with makeshift houses, random street vendors, cows and dogs and uncollected garbage. The contrast between what lies outside the gate and what is inside could not be greater. The gate separates the inside of the College from its outside. Indeed, according to a teacher at the College, 'there was no need to build such a massive gate … it was built largely in order to erect a larger and clearer border between the College and the community that had grown up around the campus'. As the city has encroached upon the College, the Board of Governors made a conscious decision to differentiate the College from the city. The gate thus serves the function of border protection, guarded around the clock, with no unauthorized person allowed in. Indeed, the guards wear military-like uniform and take a great deal of satisfaction in the role they have been asked to play.

For those who live and work in the immediate vicinity of the campus, the gate is, paradoxically, also a source of great deal of pride. Some identify their address by referring to the gate. Indeed the gate has become something of tourist site, where the visitors from nearby villages come to admire the great building that it is assumed to be. Standing outside the gate, visitors use the phrase, 'shandar hai' (stunning/magnificent/fabulous/terrific/imposing) to marvel at its beauty. The demeanor of the visitors (and potential parents) change markedly once they are allowed to go through the gate and into the campus. To be allowed in past the gate is regarded as a significant achievement, of someone whose status has been recognized not only by the College but also the broader community. According to a parent who was considering a number of schools for his only child, 'once I passed the gate, my mind was made up. I wanted to send my boy to Ripon'. In this sense, the gate is not only a physical structure, it also has a social meaning. It evokes a particular sensibility and sense of belongingness.

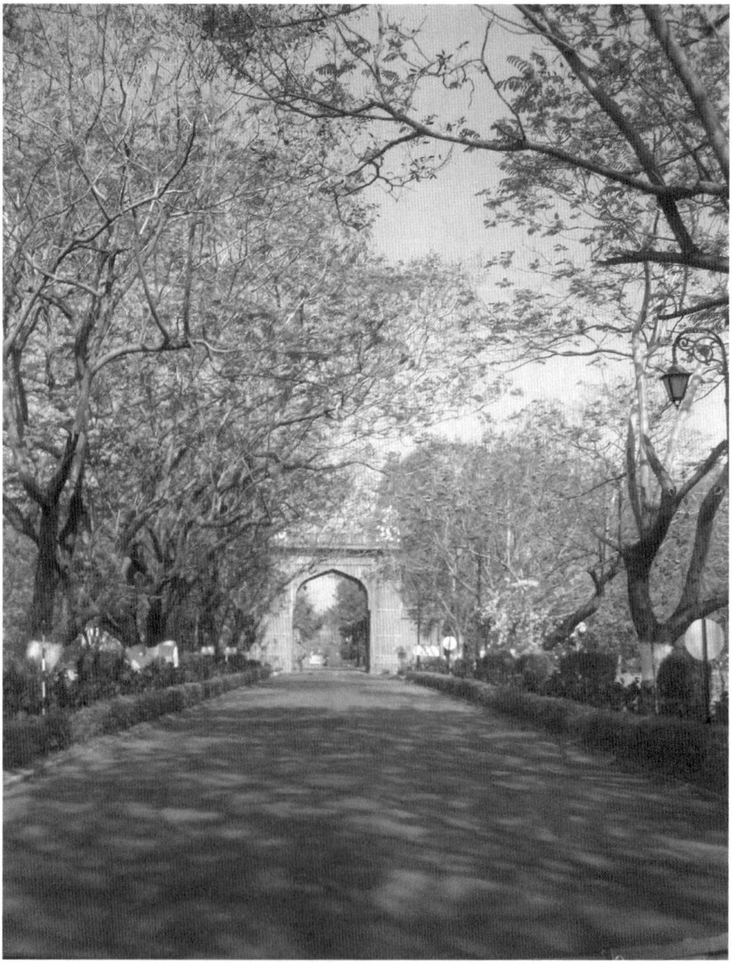

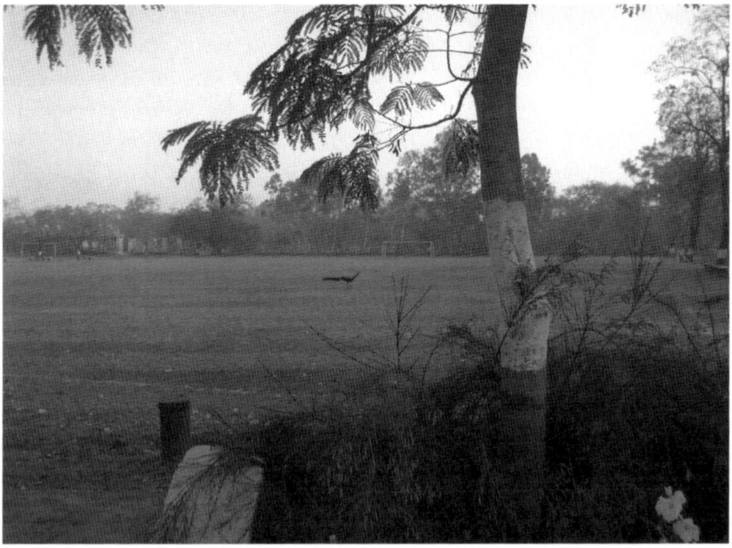

The social aesthetics surrounding the gate is enhanced by the tree-lined vista that leads to the main building of the College and the vast playing fields visible from outside the gate. This aesthetics is further elaborated by two structures of considerable significance: a disused plane donated to the College by the Indian Air Force and a disused tank donated by the Indian Army. Both are strategically positioned within meters of the gate to communicate the College's close links with the Indian power elite. From outside the gate, the plane and the tank are only partially visible, generating a sense of wonder and admiration. While for those inside the campus, they embody the College's commitment to Indian nationalism, evoking in students a sense of patriotism. They also suggest that the College prepares its students for national leadership, their capacity to defend the nation in times of need.

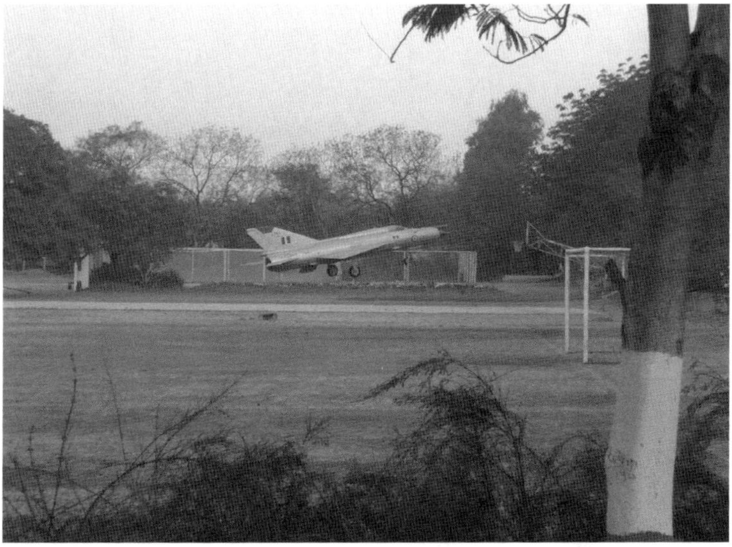

The plane and the tank also signify the close connection that the College has traditionally had with the Rajput and Maratha communities. Indeed, the College was originally established for the sons of chiefs of these communities—the original donors of the College. Rajputs in particular were known for their bravery and courage, and military leadership, and the College was established to work with the British to secure both their interests. The military artifacts thus do a great deal of symbolic work in reinforcing the sensory perceptions about the importance of Rajputs in the College's history. Arguably they are part of a cultural politics that leads many at the College to regard it as a school that is built around Rajput traditions, which treats preferentially those students and staff who belong to them. In this sense, the plane and the tank imply a particular understanding of the nation, in the construction and development of which the Rajputs are assumed to have played in a major role.

The Temple

Although Ripon College has always been committed to a secular education, religion plays an important role in its cultural life. Rare for a public school in the British tradition, a Hindu temple and a Muslim mosque are located on the campus, equidistant from the main building. The temple was built with funds provided by the Rajput and Maratha donors of the College, while the local Muslim aristocracy built the mosque. Each community had insisted that the College should not ignore the importance of the student's spiritual development, regarding this as particularly important for the boarders. For the British headmasters and teachers, the Hindu temple and a Muslim mosque exemplified their deference to local cultural traditions while the parents felt that their children were able to practice established rituals as required by their religions.

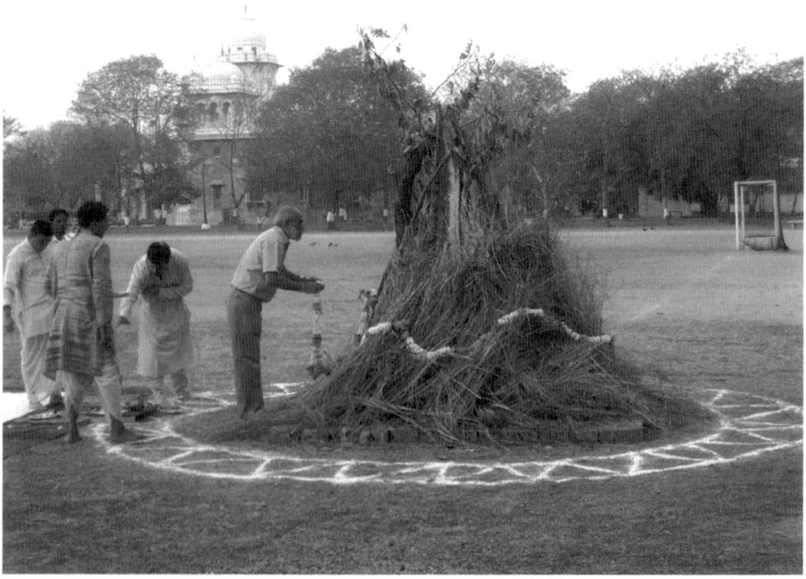

After the partition of India in 1947, the number of Muslim students declined at Ripon College. More recently, as the Hindu communities have become wealthier and more dominant throughout India, the College is left with very few Muslim students. Consequently, while the mosque is not abandoned, it is used sparsely. In contrast, the temple has become the heart of Ripon College. Many regard it as its spiritual center. It is widely used by teachers and students alike. At times of major festivals, such as Diwali and Holi, elaborate ceremonies are held in and around the temple. A number of teachers and students visit the temple every morning to say their prayers—Aarti (a Hindu religious ritual of worship). The College has appointed a senior priest and a number of assistants to provide students spiritual guidance. Student visits to the temple are frequent, especially around the time of examinations. According to a student, 'the temple is very important to me. It gives me peace of mind. I find it comforting to know it is there'.

Although Ripon College is committed to secular education, the cultural practices around the temple indicate that its secularism is now filtered through the role that the Hindu icons and practices play is the formation of its social aesthetics. For many boarding students in particular, the temple represents a link to their family and their broader community. Other students regard the temple as a sanctuary, not only a place of worship but also a point of reference for the performance of their identity. The students often bow as they go past the temple in a display of their sense of belonging to a larger universe. The College has recognized the importance of the temple in defining its imaginary of the nation. Invariably, it thus takes international visitors to the College to a ceremony at the temple in an attempt to display 'Indian culture'. The visitors are left with an impression that the Hindu ceremony illustrates some essence of India. This further reinforces the sense the students have of the emerging and perhaps hegemonic cultural construction of India as a nation—secular but predominantly Hindu. In this way, the temple plays an important role in the social aesthetics of the College both in relation to the significance that the students and staff attach to it in their everyday life but also with respect to the national meaning and significance it has for them.

The Lake

Among other locations that are important for an understanding of the social aesthetics of Ripon College, are two lakes on the campus. These lakes were built only recently but have quickly become a place around which the institutional life of the College is now performed. The official reason for constructing the lake was to conserve water. Imbued with an environmental sensibility, it was the students who first suggested the idea, arguing that the lakes would not only help conserve water on the campus but also contribute to its beautification. According to the Principal, the students insisted that the lakes would lead 'to the greening of the campus … helping to ensure that the playing fields were green throughout the year and not only during the rainy season'. The construction of the lakes became a major project for senior students at the College—as an expression of their commitment to an environmentalism that is now widely supported among the Indian middle class, especially among the young (Bhagat 2012).

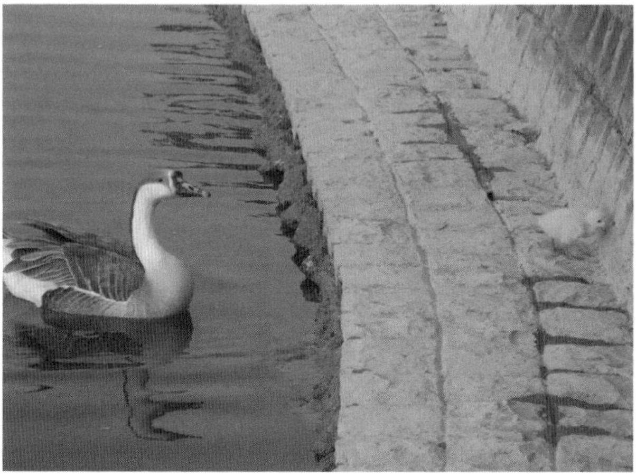

In the end, two lakes were built on the campus, one that continues to have a largely instrumental function of circulating water, while the other—the larger lake—has acquired a more important social and aesthetic role. It has been beautifully landscaped with shrubs, small patios and benches from which to admire its beauty. The lake is situated right next to a large newly built auditorium, with a large lawn between the two sites. The lawn is used to hold various receptions and functions next to the lake. The lake houses ducks, geese and swans, and is stocked with fish. The students are encouraged to learn the art of fishing at the lake. The water in the lake has attracted birds that had not been seen on the campus for years. Such is its appeal that a security guard has had to be positioned by the lake to ensure that it is not misused or vandalized. In this sense, the lake has at once many functions: cultural, environmental, pedagogic and aesthetic.

The aesthetics of the lakes has not only attracted those inside the College but also those in the broader community. The fountains and the lights that surround the lake have added to its visual possibilities, leading many alumni of the College to hold parties, wedding receptions and other functions by the lake, especially during the hot summer evenings in India's central planes. In a city whose main river has almost totally dried up, and in a country in which water has considerable cultural and religious significance, the lake has acquired a social status that the students who had proposed it had never envisaged. It has become a community-wide resource, as well as a source of revenue for the College. The College uses the best visual representations of the lake to advertise its beauty both nationally and internationally. For students, the attraction of the lake lies in 'the romance of living and learning at Ripon College', as well as a place that reinforces the College's social status and distinction.

Discussion

Social aesthetics, MacDougall maintains, is 'both the backdrop and product of everyday life', and is structured around the landscape, everyday rituals and key places of meeting. Far from being obscure or illusory, social aesthetics is 'both very obvious and highly dispersed through a wide range of cultural phenomenon' (MacDougall 2006, p. 30). This view of social aesthetics is helpful in capturing the ways in which Ripon College has marshaled its major sites to pattern the sensory experiences of its students and staff. Each of the sites—main building, the gate, the temple and the lake—have become places where the students and staff develop their sense of connectivity to Ripon College, as well as emotional attachment of its traditions. They perform a major role in the processes of social production at the College, helping to develop a sense of community. They enable the formation of aesthetic patterns, composed of objects and actions, along with relations of power and authority.

The discussion in the previous sections of this chapter amply demonstrates the efficacy of MacDougall's insights on social aesthetics—as well their applicability for understanding the ways in which Ripon College engenders sensory patterning in the experiences of students and staff. For example, it is clear that student experiences of the rituals around the temple are a product of the sensory environment constructed by the school. These sensory patterns have profound effects in creating the student's sense of belongingness to both their school—as well as their religious community. The sensory significance of the tank and the plane lies in the patriotism and other mass sentiments they generate. The gate is an expression of a more generalized power, defining the borders of the community to which the student and staff belong. As MacDougall (2007, p. 22) argues a 'fuller understanding of the social role of aesthetics may thus benefit from studies of nationalism, ethnicity, warfare, religion and sectarian politics'.

While such a call is entirely appropriate, what MacDougall's analysis of social aesthetics does not, however, sufficiently acknowledge are the ways in which sensory patterns are often a product not only of what goes on *within* the College, but also how this is linked to life *outside* the College. The social aesthetics inside the College is inextricably linked to developments in its immediate environment. The students interpret the social significance of the lake, for example, not on its own terms, but against the backdrop of the contrast it underlines between the serene conditions around the lake and the noisy, dusty and crowded condition in the city. The sensory experiences that the campus invites are constantly contrasted with the lack of opportunities available elsewhere. The experiences inside and outside the gate hence do not represent two separate aesthetic realms, but a space in which the inside is at least partially experienced with an implicit understanding of what lies outside the gate.

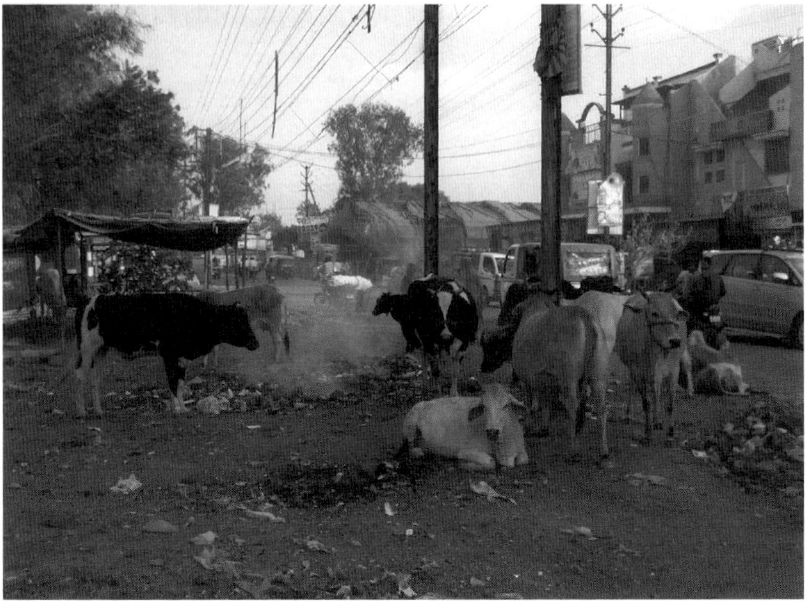

The social aesthetics of Ripon College are thus filtered through a relationality that involves a contrast between its facilities and those that the students experience in the city, and perhaps imagine exist at other schools. In this sense, the boundaries of Ripon College are not as absolute as might be imagined. What this suggests is that the students and staff do not experience the various sites, practices and routines at the College in the same way. Their sensory engagement is a product of their past experiences, their social location within the College, and their relationship to forces—local, national and global—outside the College. This relational view of social aesthetics invites an interrogation of the issue of how positionality affects the cultural politics of engagement, in forging the patterns of sensory experiences, against the backdrop of factors that do not necessarily reside within the College.

The social aesthetics of elite schools, like Ripon College,—the interpretative and affective experiences of students, teachers and parents and the schools' attempts to create an environment that elicits a particular set of aesthetic responses—is produced historically and politically, in terms that are relational. Of course, this relationality is never static and is constantly evolving, partly as a result of the changing social and historical circumstances within which schools are located and partly as a result of the ways in which the schools themselves direct attention to these circumstances. So, for example, during the colonial era, the social aesthetics of elite schools were influenced by attempts to shape the aesthetic tastes and desires of students consistent with a colonial imaginary and interests. Thus the key aesthetic markers highlighted colonial traditions, eliciting a positive response towards colonial artifacts and symbols, undermining indigenous traditions. Similarly during the nationalist postcolonial era, a new imaginary, some of the symbols of nationalist struggle against colonialism became prominent, with the signs of excessive colonial triumphalism deliberatively sidelined. In the current era of globalization, the signs and symbols of elite schools that constitute their social aesthetics have been transformed, expressing new values and aspirations of the new transnational elite class (Sklair 2001). However, this transformation is context specific, and differs markedly across various sites.

References

Bhagat, C. (2012). *What young India wants: A voice for change*. New Delhi: Rupa & Co.

MacDougall, D. (2006). *The corporeal image: Film, ethnography and the senses.* Princeton: Princeton University Press.

MacDougall, D. (2007). The experience of colour. *The Senses and Society, 2*(1), 5–26.

Sklair, L. (2001) *The transnational capitalist class*. Oxford: Blackwell.

Srivastava, S. (1998). *Constructing post-colonial India: National character and the Doon School.* London: Routledge.

Fazal Rizvi is Professor in Global Studies in Education, The University of Melbourne, Emeritus Professor, University of Illinois, Research Fellow, Australia India Institute, The University of Melbourne. His more recent research and teaching is located in the areas of education, public policy and global studies. He has a strong international reputation in a number of academic areas, including racism and multicultural education, Australia-Asia relations, models of educational policy research, theories of globalization and international education and contemporary youth cultures. His latest jointly authored books is Globalizing Education Policy (Routledge 2009); translated as Politcaseducativas en unmundoglobalizado (Morata Press 2012). Recent co-edited books are Globalizing Education Policy (N.S.S.E. 2009) and Geographies of Power, Geometries of Power: Higher Education in the twenty-first Century (Routledge 2008).

Visual Essay: Histories

Johannah Fahey

Old & New Globalizations

Time present and time past together forge time future. Founded in an earlier globalizing world where the historical forces of capitalism and colonialism created connectivity and circulation, in today's globalizing world the past is ever present in these elite schools, but so too is an unfolding future. A pair of lions, symbolizing the strength of the British Empire, and a pair of guardian dogs, Chinese symbols of protection, forms a confluence of negotiated past and present globalizing influences. An educator from the Empire, fluent in Chinese, travels to Hong Kong to tutor at Cathedral College while nowadays students from this same school broaden their horizons by travelling to other elite schools in India. Indo-Saracenic stylings, a marriage between Mughal, Gothic, Neoclassical and Art Deco architecture, ushered in the new era of the British Raj, and today that very heritage becomes a means by which Ripon College marks out its identity in a nationalizing elite school market. At the Lefkos Academy in Cyprus mid-nineteenth century standardized rules, circulated from public schools in England, determined the disciplined play of football from the school's very founding. Ersatz British battlements overshadow disciplined student cadets standing in formation under the Barbadian sun. These Barbadian cadets are observed by Chinese labors hired to rebuild the new language building where Mandarin will be taught. At Founders the original school building, which flies the Indigenous Australian flag during Reconciliation Week, is a reminder of the vestiges of colonialism sited amongst renovations for the future. At the Caledonian School, old and new, the past and the present, literally pass each other by. While at Straits School contemporary globalizing circuits of consumerism, epitomized by a 7-Eleven convenience store and an ATM machine, are situated at the very heart of the school.

J. Fahey (✉)
Monash University, Melbourne, Australia
e-mail: johannah.fahey@monash.edu

J. Fahey et al. (eds.), *In the Realm of the Senses,* Cultural Studies and Transdisciplinarity in Education, DOI 10.1007/978-981-287-350-7_13

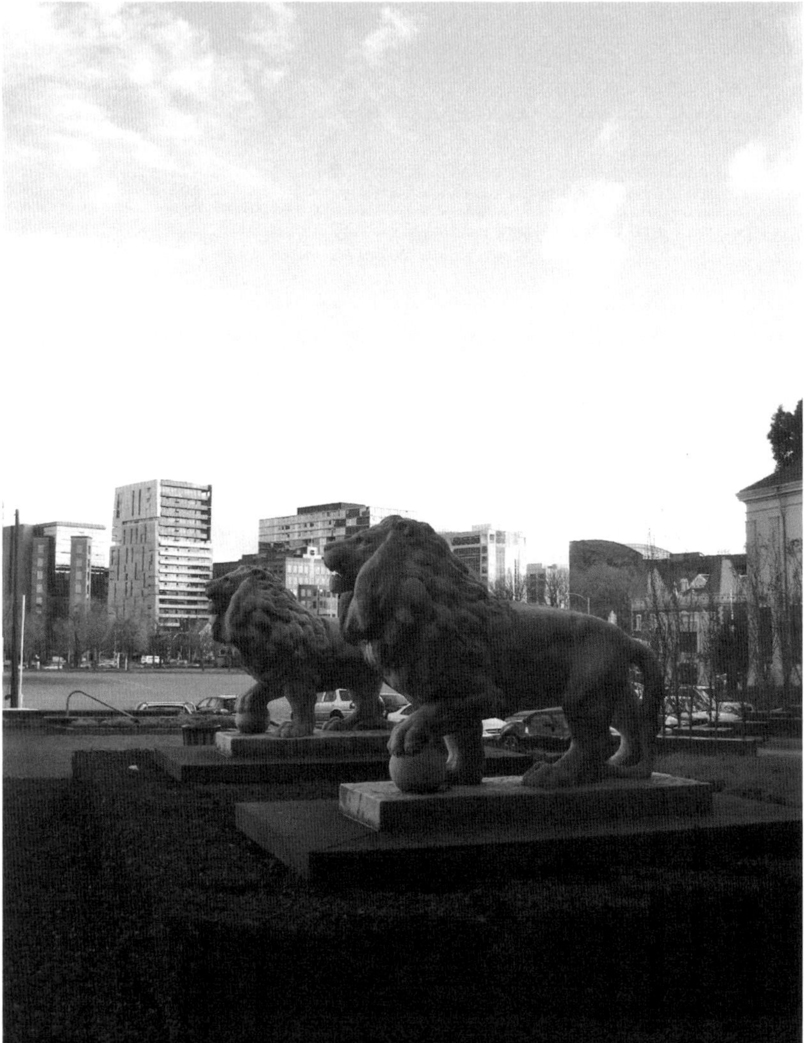

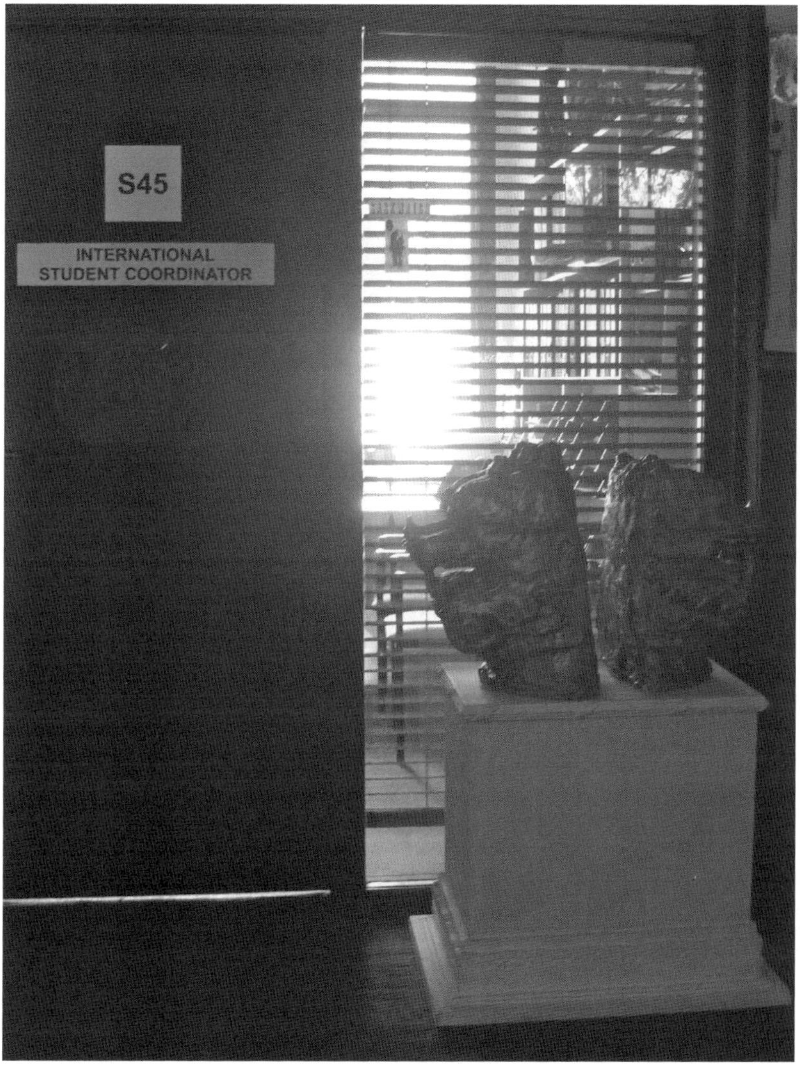
S45
INTERNATIONAL
STUDENT COORDINATOR

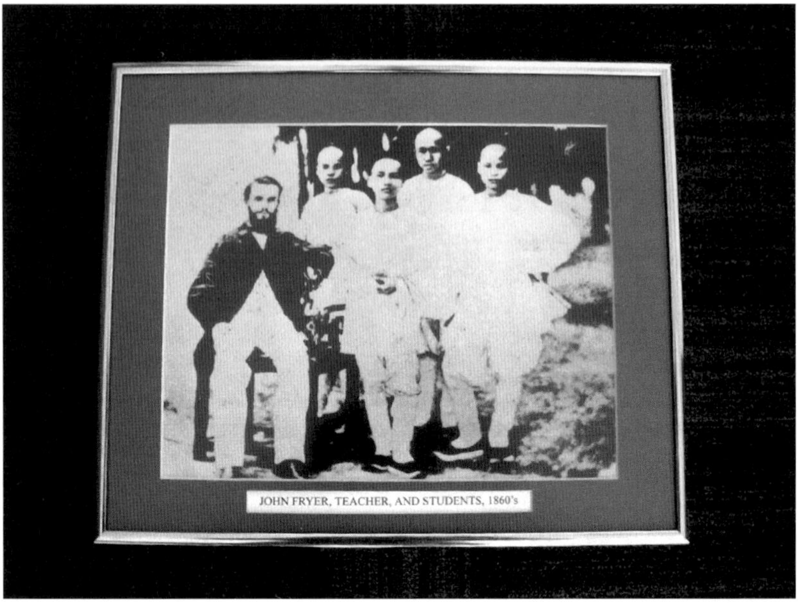
JOHN FRYER, TEACHER, AND STUDENTS, 1860's

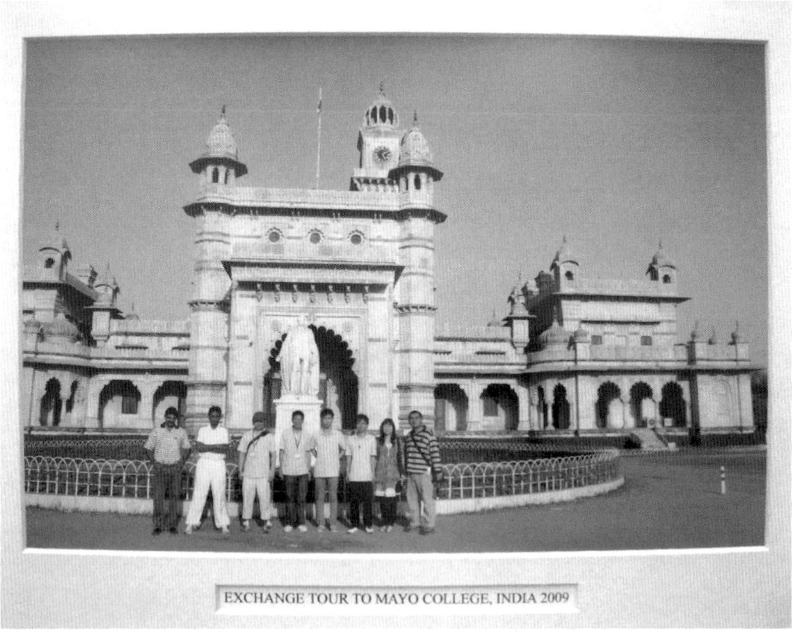
EXCHANGE TOUR TO MAYO COLLEGE, INDIA 2009

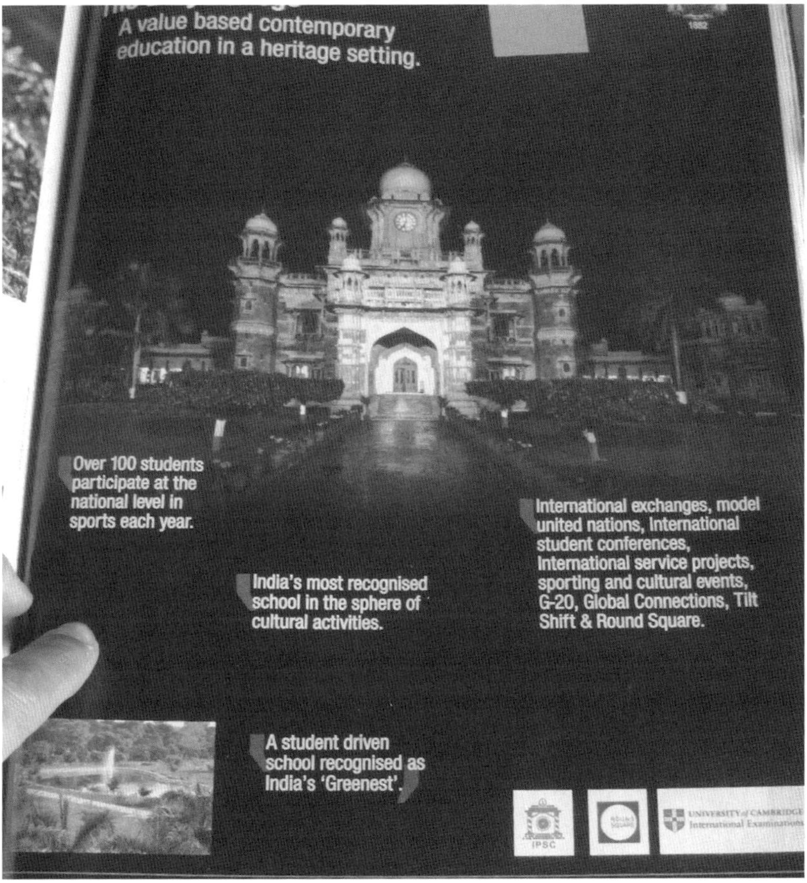
A value based contemporary
education in a heritage setting.
Over 100 students participate at the national level in sports each year.
India's most recognised school in the sphere of cultural activities.
International exchanges, model united nations, International student conferences, International service projects, sporting and cultural events, G-20, Global Connections, Tilt Shift & Round Square.
A student driven school recognised as India's 'Greenest'.
IPSC
UNIVERSITY of CAMBRIDGE
International Examinations

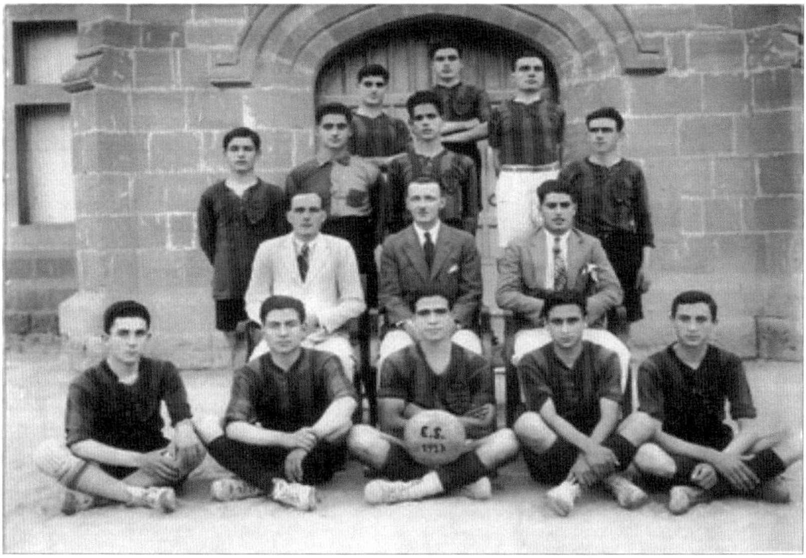

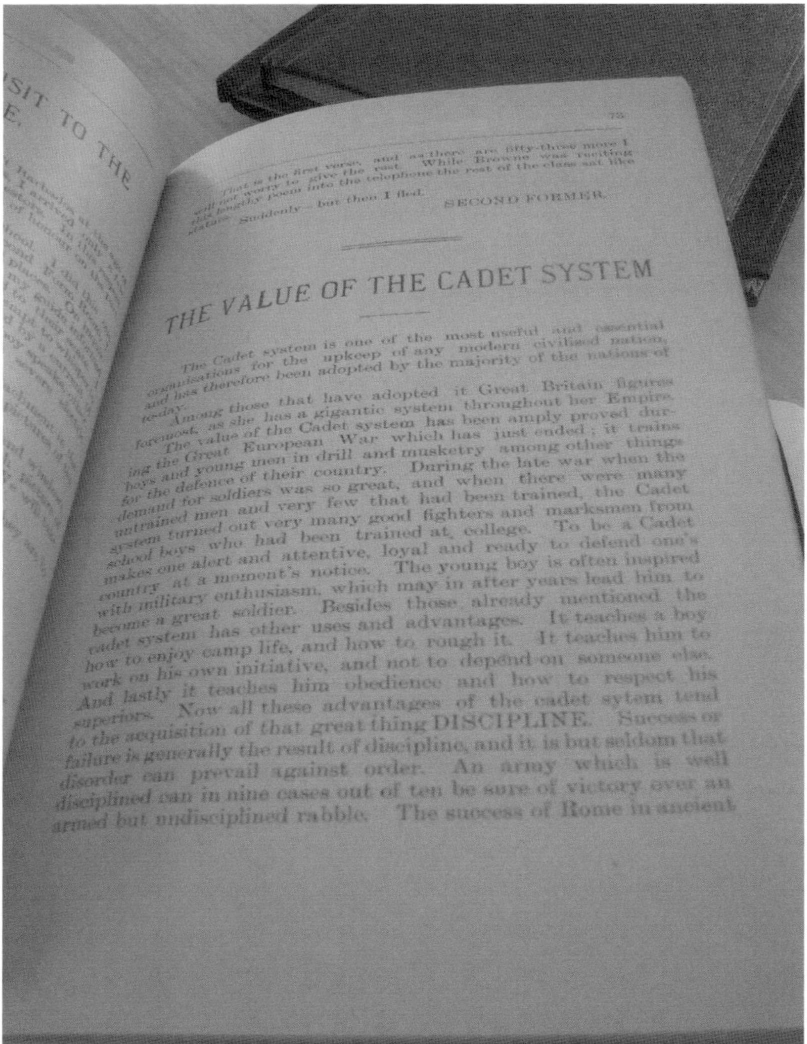

73

That is the first verse, and as there are fifty-three more I will not worry to give the rest. While Browne was reciting this lengthy poem into the telephone the rest of the class sat like statues. Suddenly—but then I fled.

SECOND FORMER.

THE VALUE OF THE CADET SYSTEM

The Cadet system is one of the most useful and essential organisations for the upkeep of any modern civilised nation, and has therefore been adopted by the majority of the nations of to-day.

Among those that have adopted it Great Britain figures foremost, as she has a gigantic system throughout her Empire.

The value of the Cadet system has been amply proved during the Great European War which has just ended; it trains boys and young men in drill and musketry among other things for the defence of their country. During the late war when the demand for soldiers was so great, and when there were many untrained men and very few that had been trained, the Cadet system turned out very many good fighters and marksmen from school boys who had been trained at college. To be a Cadet makes one alert and attentive, loyal and ready to defend one's country at a moment's notice. The young boy is often inspired with military enthusiasm, which may in after years lead him to become a great soldier. Besides those already mentioned the cadet system has other uses and advantages. It teaches a boy how to enjoy camp life, and how to rough it. It teaches him to work on his own initiative, and not to depend on someone else. And lastly it teaches him obedience and how to respect his superiors. Now all these advantages of the cadet sytem tend to the acquisition of that great thing DISCIPLINE. Success or failure is generally the result of discipline, and it is but seldom that disorder can prevail against order. An army which is well disciplined can in nine cases out of ten be sure of victory over an armed but undisciplined rabble. The success of Rome in ancient

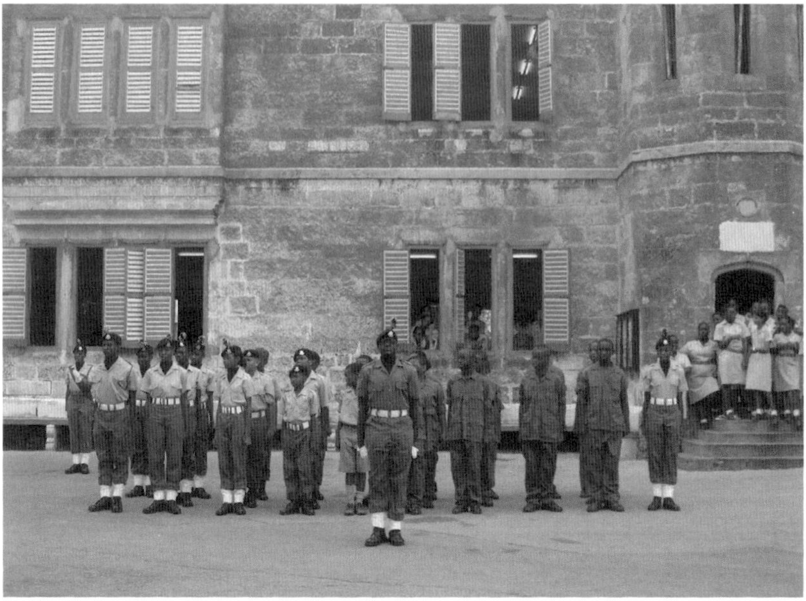

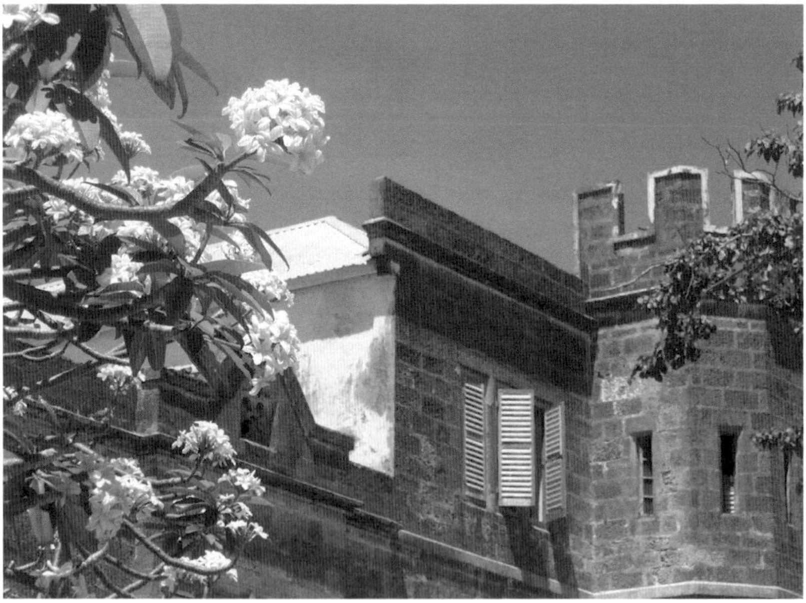

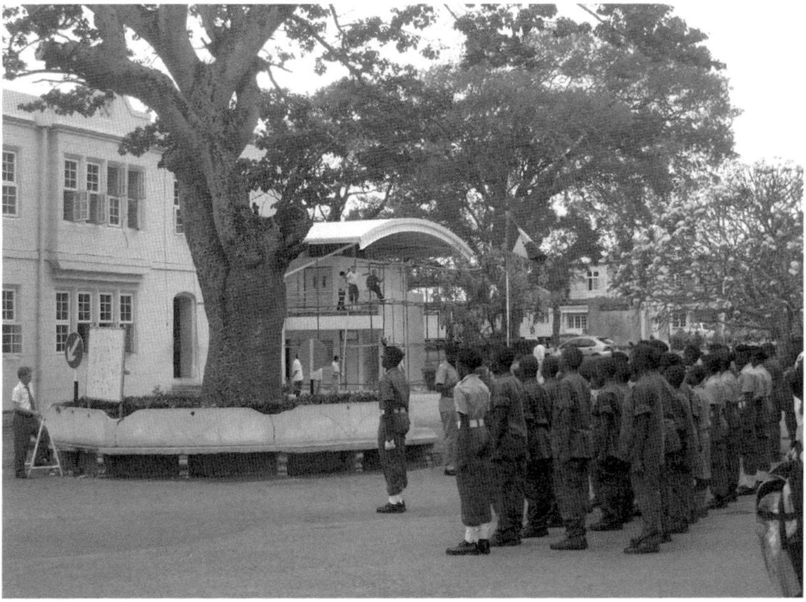

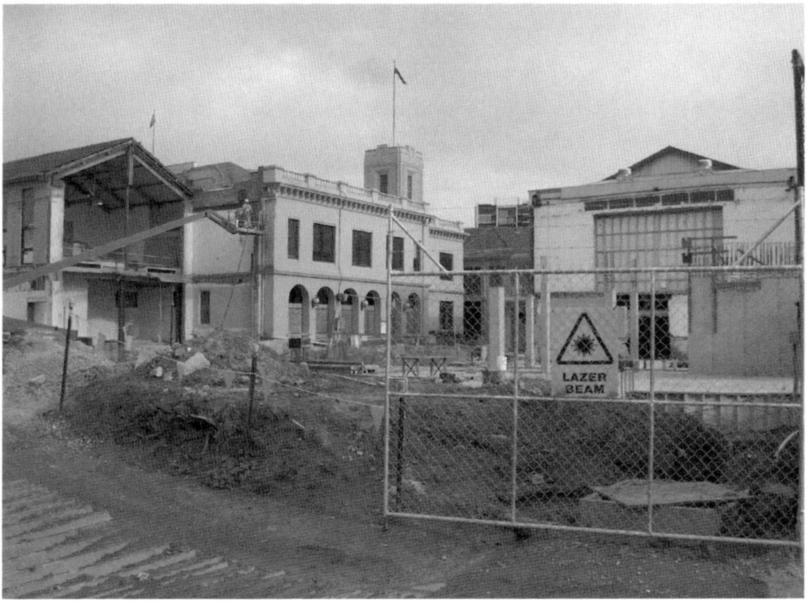
LAZER
BEAM

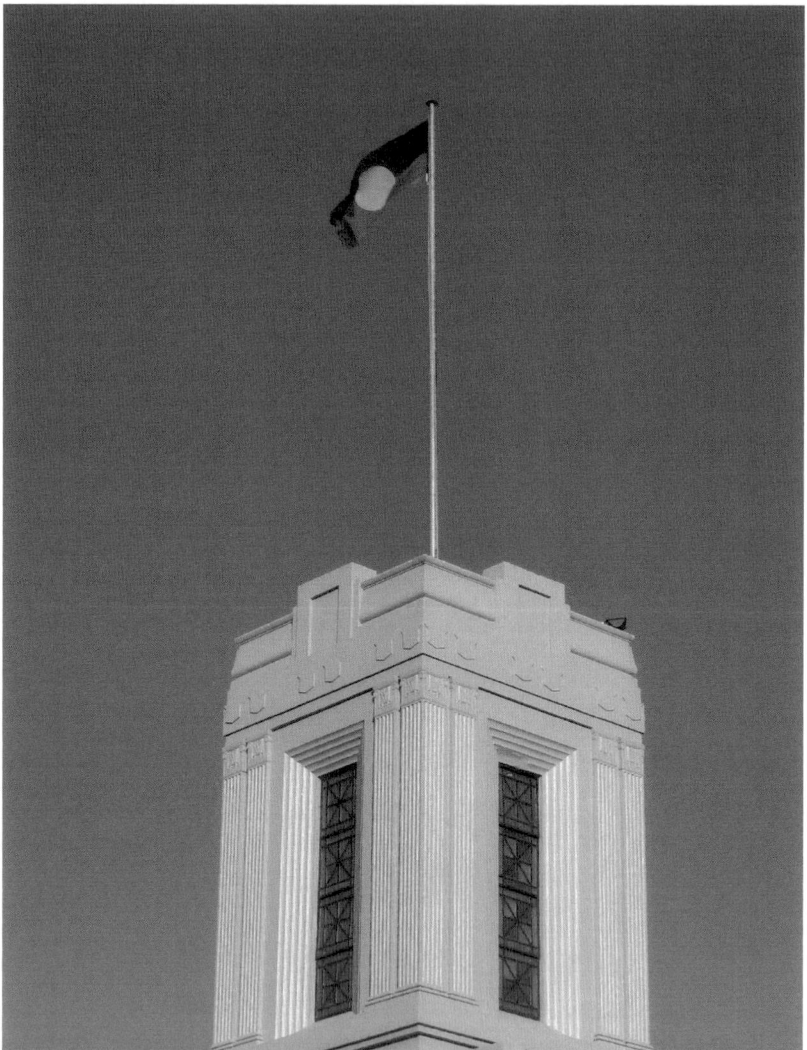

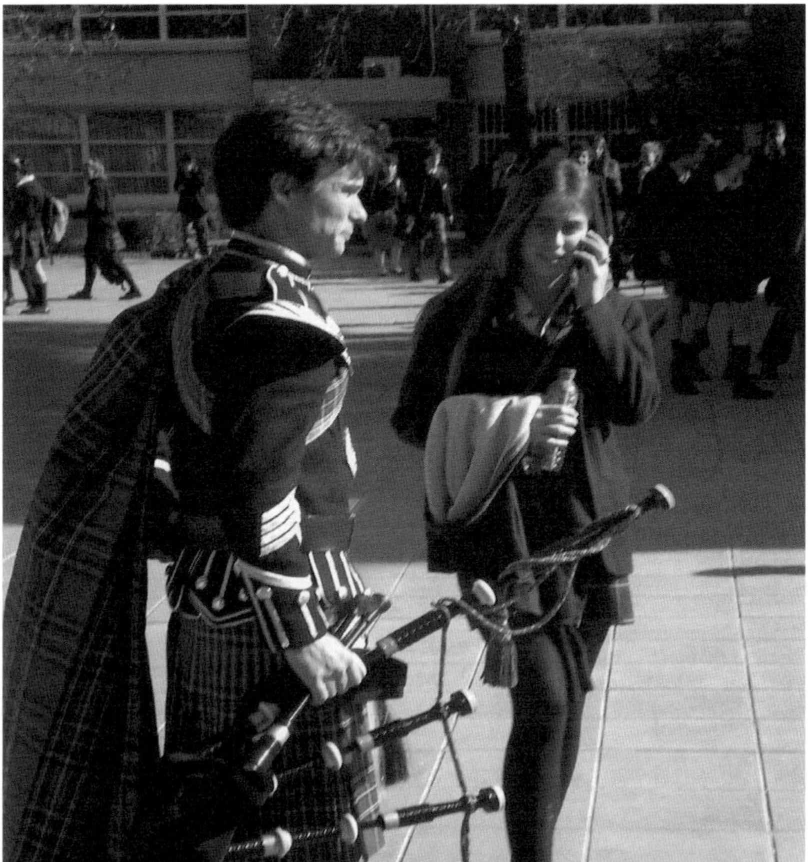

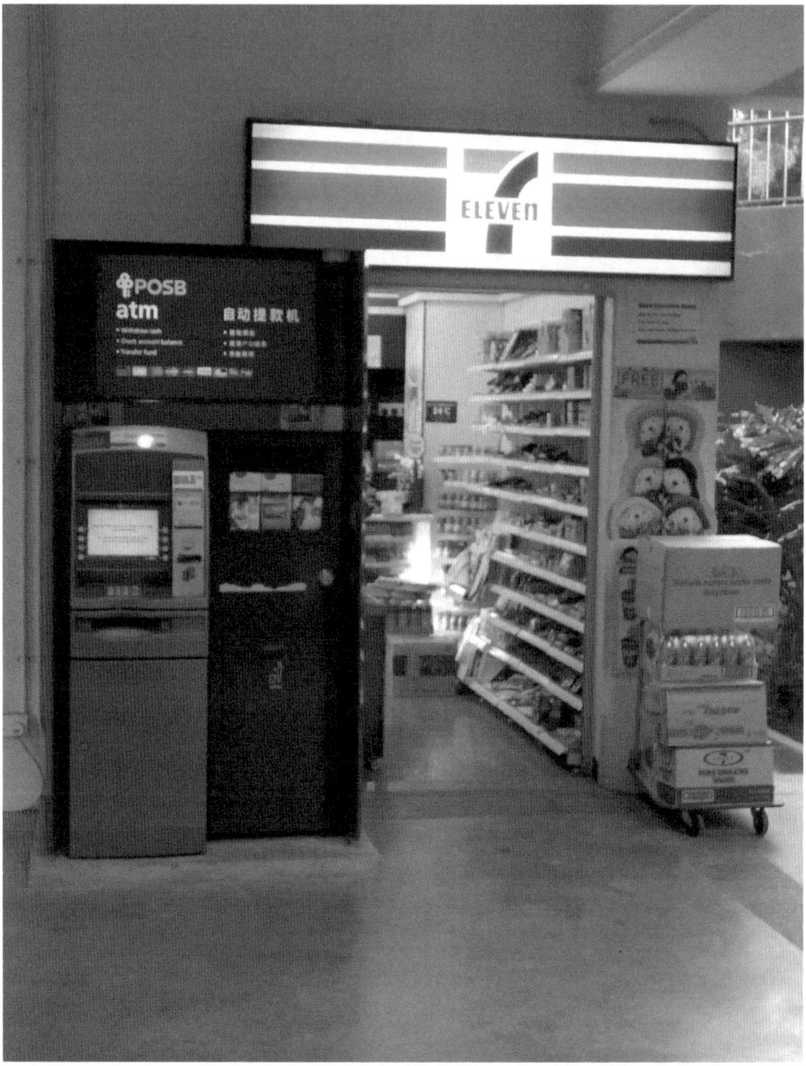

Johannah Fahey is Senior Research Fellow in the Faculty of Education at Monash University, Australia. Her research interests are located in the areas of education and global studies, and are informed by her expertise in cultural studies. She has a national and international reputation in the areas of intersectionality (gender, race and class), and cultural globalization and mobilities. She is the co-editor of Globalizing the Research Imagination (Routledge 2009); and co-author/author of Haunting the Knowledge Economy (Routledge 2006) and David Noonan: Before and Now (Thames & Hudson 2004). She has also published in many eminent international journals and edited books. She is the leading Research Fellow on the international team conducting the research project called Elite independent schools in globalising circumstances: a multi-sited global ethnography.

Vignette: The Touch of Class

Howard Prosser

What does privilege feel like? It is hard to put a finger on. I can only offer my own sense of feeling included at the Argentine school community in which I conducted my fieldwork.

The Caledonian School was extremely welcoming of my presence and only on a few occasions did I ever feel as though I was met with suspicion. This says much about the school culture as well as the way that trusted members of its community facilitated my research.

Access to elite social spaces always requires a vouched invitation. For this reason the privilege of being there allowed me to get a feel for privilege.

The feel of privilege, the touch of class, is one that can only be understood in specific contexts. What is being touched in an elite school is fairly everyday—walls, door handles, pens, computers, hands. Such things would probably not be thought extraordinary by those in the school or even outside it. Throughout Argentina almost everyone comes into contact with these things. Even laptops are now de rigueur in all public schools.

It is how and why these everyday things are used that determines privilege and eliteness. Everyday things animate social relations by creating patterned interaction. To handle such things is to touch class.

So, privilege feels like the red plastic tray collected nonchalantly from a pile as I queue alongside teachers and students to select my lunch from a large and almost self-replenishing buffet of food. The tray no doubt feels different to the men and women workers of the private catering company employed to arrange the lunch each school day. They stack them then wash them along with the cutlery and crockery and clean the hall once the lunch bell has rung. Their lunchtime, which I never saw, is different.

Privilege feels like the handle to the school doors or gates as security guards buzz me in without a word. They know me; I am not a threat. The door handle feels different to those that aren't admitted. But those people would not likely get to touch the gate: they understand that they are out of place in the school's surveilled street. The door probably feels different to the security guards that control it. They are not opening it as part of the school's educational mission; they keep it closed because

H. Prosser (✉)
Monash University, Melbourne, Australia
e-mail: howard.prosser@monash.edu

J. Fahey et al. (eds.), *In the Realm of the Senses,* Cultural Studies and Transdisciplinarity in Education, DOI 10.1007/978-981-287-350-7_14

the wealth that exists behind it feels threatened by an unstable society. Their job is protecting privilege without experiencing it for themselves.

Privilege feels like Astroturf burning my leg's skin as I overzealously play football with members of the school staff—from the principal to the security guards—each week. When we play a few times on the manicured grass of the school's playing fields these burns are avoided. Tackles slide smoothly. At other Argentine schools such rough and tumble occurs on concrete *patios* as children chase footballs, which are sometimes tennis balls, around a crowded space. Their skin is bruised and scabbed from the bitumen. They, like us, emulate the virtuosity of their sporting heroes as the ball hits their feet. Their skin feels the same type of fabric as they reveal their team's strip, especially the sky-blue-and-white striations of the national team. Those kids probably play better than us; but under our feet the ground is more kempt.

Privilege feels like the polyester back seats of a *remise* that takes me between campuses at the school. It feels like the biro with which I sign the receipt or the money with which I pay. They feel different to the steering wheel of the car or the change given back to me. They are different from the vinyl seats of radio taxis or the buses most *porteños* use to get around. This car's air-conditioning cools my skin and I feel comfortable.

To be privileged is to repeatedly feel such things, caress them over and over, so that personal comfort contains inklings of social anxiety.

Privilege feels like everybody is missing out. But you're not.

Howard Prosser researches and teaches at the Faculty of Education, Monash University, Australia. He has taught history in Australian secondary schools and universities. His research interests include Social Theory, History of Ideas, and Ethnography. Most recently he has been working on a study of political culture at an elite school in Argentina.

Afterword

David MacDougall

Abstract In the Afterword, MacDougall discusses the ways in which social aesthetics has been advanced in this book by taking into account the broader contexts of class, race, gender, post-colonial history, and global society.

A prominent theme of this book is the need to place the particular social aesthetics of elite schools, and presumably other 'total' institutions, within the broader contexts of class, race, gender, postcolonial history, and global society. This is a laudable goal and one that the book clearly advances. All of the schools described here are connected to the societies around them, and they not only contribute to local and national power structures but reflect them in their own ideology and internal organization. As conditions vary from country to country, so the individual characteristics of the schools vary, but as the authors of Chapter Ten "The Visual Field of Barbadian Elite Schooling: Towards Postcolonial Social Aesthetics" point out, there are many visible resemblances and parallels among them in their rituals, emblems, and deployment of physical objects. Yet while visual evidence is important, the social aesthetics of an institution runs deeper than the visible, involving not only the other senses but also the symbolic systems and behavioral dispositions that the anthropologist Ivo Strecker and his colleagues have called 'rhetoric culture'. There may be no single, overarching visible social aesthetic capable of encompassing this diversity.

Ethnography and social analysis call for varied strategies and, as Aaron Koh points out in Chapter Five "The (semiotics of) Social Aesthetics in an Elite School in Singapore: An Ethnographic Study", this has made the visual media useful contributors to contemporary anthropological research. At the same time it is apparent that some strategies are more suitable for some tasks than others. Film, video, and still photography are good at communicating the specific instance in its fine detail and expressing the nuances of interpersonal relations, but they are not so good at the more abstract work of generalization, comparison, and propounding hypotheses, conclusions, and propositional statements. I would argue that unlike written texts these media lack a *propositional register*, although they can develop complex

D. MacDougall (✉)
Australian National University, Canberra, Australia
e-mail: david.macdougall@anu.edu.au

J. Fahey et al. (eds.), *In the Realm of the Senses*, Cultural Studies and Transdisciplinarity in Education, DOI 10.1007/978-981-287-350-7_15

themes and interrelationships in their structure. They may be somewhat better at explanation, but chiefly because by showing how something happens they can frequently show us why it happens. We must therefore be careful to distinguish the most appropriate methods for exploring social aesthetics from the methods better suited to theorizing about it.

I have focused most of my attention on the affective and material aspects of the social aesthetics field and in identifying the existence of such a field, using video as a primary research tool. This is an appropriate job for ethnography. It can be approached directly through participant-observation, through the experiences of newcomers learning the customs of the institutions they enter, through their testimonies and memories, and through comparisons of one institution with another. We need to extend this, however, by examining specific instances in which decision-making has been determined by aesthetic concerns as much as by economics, politics, class, and ideology. This is a task that visual media cannot accomplish alone. It will require other ethnographic tools as well as written analysis.

Such an analysis will need to avoid the reductionism of mistaking academic classification for understanding. Roland Barthes drew our attention to the varied 'mythologies' that operate in contemporary society, but he was always careful to caution us against allowing what he called the 'third' or 'obtuse' meaning to be subsumed by language, or, I would suggest, by critical theory. 'What the obtuse meaning disturbs, sterilizes, is metalanguage (criticism)' (Barthes 1977, p. 61). This resonates with Lucien Castaing-Taylor's protest against the 'linguification' of film, and by extension many other aspects of society (Taylor 1996). There will always be an irreducible core of social experience that cannot be relegated to information or symbolic meaning. In studying social aesthetics it is therefore important to understand its complexities *in situ* rather than reducing it to a set of abstractions. Further, as I have argued elsewhere, considering specific aesthetic features of a society in too great isolation runs the risk of making them appear too prominent, when this is not at all the experience of those for whom the social aesthetics field is an intricately woven tapestry in which rituals, individual habits, and material objects are all enmeshed.

The study of elite schools through the lens of aesthetics is of course only a beginning. If aesthetic factors are important in such institutions and are to be taken seriously in social research, how are the principles that are uncovered to be applied to other social groups? For a start, what can we learn from such relatively hermetic communities as religious orders, military organizations, and ships at sea? If aesthetics is a significant force in these communities, it is perhaps equally at play in the life of more porous and heterogeneous institutions: corporations, financial institutions, universities, intelligence services, and government agencies. If that is so, what part has it played historically? Some have pointed to its role in the maintenance of nation states.[1] In Chapter One "Introduction: Local Classes, Global Influences—Considerations on the Social Aesthetics of Elite Schools", Johannah Fahey and her colleagues make a case for the role of aesthetics in the expansion of the British Empire.

[1] See, for example, Theweleit 1989 and Groys 1992.

Its expansion was the result of many forces, not least of which was the pursuit of profits and jobs, to which must be added the pressure of ideas about race and religion, and militancy itself. In each of these areas aesthetics may have played a part, but how, and in which, and to what degree, will require further examination. It is in pursuing such larger questions that I believe the potential of studying social aesthetics now lies.

I hope this book will encourage further debate and study of the subject.

References

Barthes, R. (1977). *Image-music-text: Essays* (Selected and trans: S. Heath). London: Fontana.

Groys, B. (1992). *The total art of Stalinism: Avant-Garde, aesthetic dictatorship, and beyond* (trans: Charles Rougle). Princeton: Princeton University Press.

Taylor, L. (1996). Iconophobia: How anthropology lost it at the movies. *Transition, 6*(1), 64–88.

Theweleit, K. (1989). *Male bodies: Psychoanalyzing the white terror*. Minneapolis: University of Minnesota Press.

David MacDougall is an ethnographic filmmaker and writer on visual anthropology and documentary cinema. Born in the USA of American and Canadian parents, he has lived in Australia since 1975. He was educated at Harvard University and the University of California at Los Angeles. His first film To *Live with Herds* won the Grand Prix "Venezia Genti" at the Venice Film Festival in 1972. Soon after this, he and his wife Judith MacDougall produced the Turkana Conversations trilogy of films on semi-nomadic camel herders of northwestern Kenya. With Judith MacDougall, he then directed or co-directed a number of films on indigenous communities in Australia. In 1997 he began conducting a study of the Doon School in northern India. This resulted in five films: *Doon School Chronicles* (2000), *With Morning Hearts* (2001), *Karam in Jaipur* (2001), *The New Boys* (2003), and *The Age of Reason* (2004). His latest film, *Gandhi's Children* (2008), concerns a shelter for homeless children in New Delhi. MacDougall writes regularly on documentary and ethnographic cinema and is the author of *Transcultural Cinema* (Princeton University Press, 1998) and *The Corporeal Image: Film, Ethnography, and the Senses* (Princeton, 2006).

Index

J. Fahey et al. (eds.), *In the Realm of the Senses*, Cultural Studies and Transdisciplinarity in Education, DOI 10.1007/978-981-287-350-7